Praise f(

If I Can Climb Mount Kilimanjaro, Why Can't I Brush My Teeth?

"Nan Little's determination and guts got her to the summit of Mt. Kilimanjaro and across Iowa by bike 4 times. But she generously says that all those with Parkinson's disease (PD) who exercise daily 'climb a mountain higher than Kilimanjaro' every time. Read her book to discover how a 60+ year-old grandmother turned a PD diagnosis into a prescription for exercise, filling her life with unimaginable moments.

"Be inspired as an armchair adventurer and read some of the clearest descriptions of the 'facts' of PD. As you follow Nan on her journeys, recollect your own journeys and explore the heights you achieved when you persevered to your own summits. Then give a cheer for yourself and Nan Little whose achievements are large!"

--Katherine Huseman
President, Parkinsons Creative Collective, Inc. Editor, author, The Peripatetic Pursuit of Parkinson Disease. Lives with Parkinson's disease.

"Steve Jobs said the most important thing in life is when you realize your actions can leave a mark in the world, 'The minute you understand you can poke life and if you push in something will pop out the other side. That's maybe the most important thing.'

"When life poked Nan Little she poked back.

"Her incredibly personal story of empowerment and adventure has made her an inspirational figure in the Parkinson's disease community. Her journey takes the reader across four continents: to fishing the fabled trout streams of Montana and Idaho,

to cycling across America's heartland of Iowa, to climbing the summit of Africa's tallest mountain Kilimanjaro, to trekking Annapurna base camp in Nepal and the Inca Trail in Peru. Like any journey worth pursuing, victories are accompanied by setbacks, and lessons learned are worth sharing.

"Nan's story is a testament to what can be achieved when we tap into the power of mind and body to alter life's course."

--Jeff Broderick
Co-Founder & CEO
Beneufit, Inc.

"Delightfully humorous, heartfelt, and inspiring. This book is a must read that will inspire you to live each moment to its fullest.

"Nan is the embodiment of strength, courage, and tenacity. In this book she gives honest and raw insight into the process one goes through after being diagnosed with a neurodegenerative disease and how our biggest trial can give us our greatest life lessons."

--Brandis Gunderson
Owner: Baker to Bay Wellness Center
Kilimanjaro climber with MS

"Unlike most people with degenerative diseases, Nan lives her life squarely in the face of her Parkinson's—engaged and optimistic but realistic, as well. As she says, it's not always easy, but it is her life and the decisions belong to her alone. I applaud Nan for her courageousness in writing this book so others may learn from her mistakes, triumphs, missteps and accomplishments."

"PWPs often feel out of control of their lives; Nan grudgingly accepts what she cannot do and embraces the challenges she's capable of defeating."

--Steve Wright
Executive Director
Northwest Parkinson's Foundation

"….Nan Little is the inspiration everyone needs when dealing with something as overwhelming as a diagnosis of a disease. With her intuitive spirit and dedication to her health, husband, family and friends, Nan shows how even the most challenging obstacles life puts in front of us can be stepping-stones to something greater than we ever dreamed! Her commitment to bringing what she's learned to others who experience the same challenges has motivated and supported people with Parkinson's more than any research study, physician recommendation or hospital program.

On her own, Nan crossed America meeting with YMCA after YMCA to share her passion for living a full and rich life despite being struck with Parkinson's. Nan didn't let anything stand in the way of getting back to her former self and she shares that commitment with everyone she meets. You'll be inspired to climb new heights, achieve new milestones and reach every dream you ever had when you encounter a moment with Nan…"

--Linna Dossett
Senior Director for Healthy Living
YMCA of Greater Seattle

If I Can Climb Mount Kilimanjaro, Why Can't I Brush My Teeth?

Courage, Tenacity and Love Meet Parkinson's Disease

Nan Little

IF I CAN CLIMB MT. KILIMANJARO,

why can't I brush my teeth?

Courage, Tenacity & Love Meet Parkinson's Disease

Book Cover Design: Susie Weber
Editing: Kathy Bradley

All photos were taken by the author unless otherwise noted. Grateful acknowledgment is made to professional photographers Jeff Rennicke, JeffRennicke.com, Kevin Erdman, VideoBigwig.com, and Richard Baccus, rbaccus.com for permission to reproduce selected photos as noted.

First Edition
Printed in the United States of America
ISBN 978-1-50875-834-0 (paperback)

DEDICATION

For Doug,

Whose love fuels my courage and tenacity.

Contents

"Only those who will risk going too far
can possibly find out how far they can go."
T. S. Eliot

"All journeys outward
Are journeys inward."

Joe DiIenno

Foreword by Jay Alberts

An often repeated axiom many people hear as they make the transition from "never sick a day of my life" to a person with a neurological disease, such as Parkinson's is: *"When life gives you lemons, make lemonade."* This statement is usually a default for many as what do you say when your spouse, friend or colleague tells you they have Parkinson's disease? It is certainly more reassuring than informing your wife that you may start trolling Craigslist for potential replacements. While the statement undoubtedly has provided encouragement and facilitated a positive attitude in the face of adversity, change or challenge for many, it is a bit trite as sour lemons do not magically turn into a cool refreshing glass of lemonade with a flipping of the positive thinking switch.

A quick Google of the "best recipe for lemonade" revealed that it is quite a process to convert lemons to lemonade. Making lemonade requires the right mix of any number of sweeteners, the right amount of lemon juice (preferably squeezed from a perfect lemon) and water. Much to my surprise one must combine all the ingredients, bring it to a boil while continuously stirring and mixing while monitoring its consistency and finally, after all the sugar is dissolved and letting it cool, serve over ice, preferably in a chilled glass. Sounds like a lot of work. I will trust my thirst to the experts at Dole or Minute Maid and head to the refrigerated section of the grocery store. Ok, so lemons to lemonade is not easy for us "healthy" folks. Having Parkinson's throws a bit of wrinkle in this not so easy process as no two "lemons" or manifestations of the disease symptoms are the same, so there are no perfect recipes out there and as the disease progresses the pH of the lemons change so recipes that worked ok yesterday do not work today.

The story of Dr. Nan Little, anthropologist, advocate, mother, grandmother, wife and person with Parkinson's is not a guidebook or recipe book in how to turn lemons into lemonade, rather it is a fresh and truthful account of living with and constantly battling the disease she shares with more than 1 million other Americans and more than 4 million people worldwide. It is her account of denying the existence of lemons, hiding the lemons, fearing the lemons, throwing the lemons at her husband Doug and continually developing and testing the optimal recipe to create lemonade that was not just bearable, but provided refreshment.

It is this continual and dogged commitment to keep adjusting the recipe, while understanding at some point the lemons will be too great to overcome, that is the inspirational point of this book. To me, commitment to this process is courage and it reminds me of Harper Lee's Atticus Finch character in "*To Kill a Mockingbird*", when he tells Jem what it means to have courage "...It's when you know you are licked before you begin, but you begin anyway and see it through no matter what. You rarely win, but sometimes you do." Unfortunately, despite advances in the treatment of Parkinson's disease, there is no cure and the disease eventually wins. Some may find this last statement depressing or lacking sensitivity. I am sorry if it offends, but even those who never transition to a neurological disease will not win as we all expire at some point. Nan's story inspires all to see it through and while you may not win, you will have victories along the way.

I got to know Nan and her Craigslist addicted husband Doug in 2008 when she emailed me asking about a recent study conducted in my laboratory related to the effectiveness of "forced-exercise" in the relief of the motor symptoms associated with Parkinson's disease. Briefly, we found that exercising on a tandem cycle at relatively high pedaling rates resulted in significant improvements in the cardinal symptoms of Parkinson's disease. Nan heard about the study and emailed me and I most likely did not respond very quickly so I am convinced she sent additional emails and called me. I answered the phone that day, and she did not even have to pretend to be a real doctor. The person on the other end of the phone sounded so much like the other Parkinson's disease patients who had called previously looking for relief from this disease that steals their control over their body. As we talked I realized that this was not a woman who was looking to head directly to the refrigerated section of the neurological arsenal for Parkinson's treatment hoping a few weeks of pedaling on the bike would cure her Parkinson's. She pressed me on the details and what she could do since she did not have a tandem bike to ride. She committed to making exercise part of her lifestyle. It was then that I invited her and Doug to pedal across Iowa that next summer with the Pedaling For Parkinson's team. She and Doug accepted the invitation and made the long drive to Iowa in July to ride with us. My daughter immediately unconditionally loved Nan and Doug, as long as their mini Dachshund was within arm's reach. This was the start of a treasured relationship between Nan and Doug and my family.

Nan takes you through her trials, tribulations and adventures over the past seven years as she continually tweaks the recipe. Recalling the ups and downs of the ascent of Mt. Kilimanjaro to the Inca Trail reminds me of the great books from Ed Viestur, one of the most accomplished mountaineers in North America. As Mr. Viestur so elegantly proclaims that in mountaineering, there are no short cuts to the top, Nan too relates how you cannot stop the "dancing hand" by merely shoving it in your pocket or sitting on it.

Nan has accomplished and completed more physical feats than the majority of the "neurologically normal" population. She has ridden her bike in place on the trainer in some of the most beautiful and picturesque country in the USA. I end most of my scientific talks with her pedaling her bike on a trainer in Yellowstone with Mt. Haynes in the background. When I saw that picture and asked her why she brought her trainer on their trips, she responded, "I bike so I can fish!" The feats that Nan has accomplished are impressive and a testament to her courage and tenacity and the love and support of Doug, her family and her friends. I consider myself a friend and one who may have inspired her slightly, but I think I have learned more from her than I could ever teach or tell her. What I have learned from her is that in order to battle this disease that tries to steal control of your arms and legs and fingers and messes with your cognition, you do not have to ascend a mountain or trek an ancient trail or even ride a bike across the greatest state in the Union. Rather, it is getting out of the comfortable chair of self-pity and taking that first step in the journey of fighting this disease. Whether it is lifting your foot over one rock, walking a mile or taking one more step, it is about the journey and having the courage to not give up or quit even though you may be "killing the fish...". She embodies the spirit of courage that Atticus described.

Nan and Doug have been critical in the proliferation of Pedaling For Parkinson's programs throughout the YMCA system and other health care organizations. I personally have witnessed them spend the day riding their bikes in the heat and humidity during those late July days and still have energy to talk with another person interested in Parkinson's or join me in giving a talk to support groups along the route. It is important to note that the number of attendees at these talks can be more than a hundred or as few as six or seven who may have dementia and have no idea what we are talking about. She is always willing to share her story and it is a story that is worth hearing and listening to. As Robert Frost notes, "I have miles to go before I sleep." I am confident that Nan has many more miles to travel in her relentless, yet sensible, pursuit of the best recipe to turn those sour ass lemons into lemonade.

--Jay L. Alberts, Ph.D.

Vice Chair of Health Technology Enablement, Neurological Inst. Director, Cleveland Clinic Concussion Center.
The Edward F. and Barbara A. Bell Family Endowed Chair.
Staff, Biomedical Engineering

Introduction

A full moon brilliantly illuminated Mount Kilimanjaro, casting eerie shadows on an unlikely assemblage of individuals eager to join a centipede of headlamps inching its way up the final 4,000 feet of ascent. After milling around, becoming increasingly chilled in the deepening cold, at 10:45 p.m. our group stepped on the trail. Just before we started my husband, Doug, whispered to me, "I know you can make it."

I was not sure just why I was participating in this "Empowerment Through Adventure: A Leap of Faith" journey. Perhaps I came because I had been asked to climb Mount Kilimanjaro with a group of people with neurodegenerative diseases who were determined to show the world our diseases didn't define us, and I liked meeting challenges. Companion climbers provided support for the fourteen of us living with either multiple sclerosis or Parkinson's disease. We had already spent five and a half days getting to this point on the mountain, some battling acute mountain sickness along with our chronic diseases, others easily scaling the peak.

I was the only woman with Parkinson's, and the oldest of all of us carrying the extra weight of a neurodegenerative disease. Kilimanjaro was the first mountain I had ever climbed. Attempting to reassure me before we left home, a friend had proclaimed blithely, "It's like taking a walk in the park, only at high elevation." It was not.

The next morning, July 18, 2011, I stood atop Mount Kilimanjaro, at age sixty-five years and nine months perhaps the oldest woman with Parkinson's disease to trek to the summit—unassisted—via the Machame route, or if not the oldest, certainly one of a select few.

A year later as I gazed at myself in the bathroom mirror, unable to brush my teeth in familiar up-and-down, side-to-side motions, I reached for my electric toothbrush.

My story is about finding strength to meet challenges, physical and neurological challenges that come as a result of having Parkinson's, with courage and tenacity and love.

Chapter 1. More than Lemonade

Parkinson's books tend to focus on positive aspects of having the disease. Although the negatives are all too obvious, there *are* some benefits. Designed to encourage newly diagnosed People with Parkinson's (PwPs), authors emphasize making lemonade out of lemons. Whereas an upbeat attitude makes a huge difference in both slowing disease progression and determining how PwPs are "doing," a certain lie is embedded in this approach. Having an incurable disease, whether or not it's a neurodegenerative disease like mine, is a bad deal. Prognosis, diagnosis and reality tell us that over time the disease will worsen and the patient will become increasingly debilitated, quite possibly even demented. It's not a pretty prospect. No matter what resources a person has—intellectual, physical, financial, emotional, spiritual or community-based—there is no denying that at some point the scales will tip in favor of the disease. Although the disease eventually will dominate, how soon and to what degree it does so is likely determined in some part by the PwP.

Many people claim that if you just believe, and you try hard, you can do nearly anything. They cite my story as proof. If an older woman like me can climb Mount Kilimanjaro, trek to Annapurna Base Camp, climb the Inca Trail to Machu Picchu and ride her bike across Iowa time after time, surely anyone with Parkinson's disease can get on a bike and rid themselves of their symptoms. I used to try to believe that was true until I experienced real-life stories of others with designer diseases such as mine, "designer" because they present differently in each individual. Many PwPs have tremors, some have none, some walk fluidly, others cannot pass through a doorway and on it goes. As I saw each individual experience a different version of the disease, I realized that no amount of effort would enable most people to climb mountains or possibly even walk around the block. Defining what it means to successfully cope with the disease, then, is not wholly about attitude, but attitude informs how we respond. We do have choices.

People tell me they are inspired to try harder, or to try anything at all, because they've heard my story. There are moments and even times of day when I am sure everything is going to be just fine, sometimes countered by moments and times of day when I feel like I'd like to call it game over and just wrap up the enterprise. But I keep going because I know bad times will pass and good times will return. Caveat: "Good times" are not to be confused with "disease free." Lemons cannot always be turned into lemonade.

Chapter 2. Prelude to Diagnosis

Experts claim there are seven stages of grief, the first being denial. In retrospect, I denied a problem existed for many months, even years. I blamed anomalies on advancing age or temporary flaws in my system and dismissed them as background noise. I have never been seriously ill in my life. I'm still not ill. Although I have a disease, I'm seldom sick. Possibly separating disease from illness is a coping mechanism I developed to help me give my disease a specific place in my world but not control over my life.

I wasn't the only one who denied. By January 2007 the shooting, stabbing pains and cramps in my right forearm were so severe I wasted money on an arm massager. Ruling out carpal tunnel syndrome, a neurologist claimed I had double tendonitis. My already nearly illegible handwriting deteriorated, but at least I could still write. Though many doctors weighed in on what could be causing my various symptoms, no one mentioned Parkinson's or Parkinsonism. It took over another year before I was actually diagnosed.

♪ ♪ ♪ ♪ ♪

The year 2007, the last Year Before Diagnosis, had its moments. For the last few years my husband and I have lived in a little camper van for several months while fly-fishing and visiting old friends. In the spring of 2007 we extended the trip, traveling east for Doug's fortieth college reunion. We enjoyed our 4 Fs: Fishing (in rivers from Montana to New York), Fighting (exploring Civil War battlegrounds), Friends (reconnecting with old classmates) and Family (visiting every relative in our path). Each day brought new experiences along with opportunities to connect with our personal and national pasts.

At Princeton graduation time the whole campus was turned over to Reunions as alumni returned to campus to reconnect with their formative educational roots and old friends. With bands and entertainment around each corner, people felt no compunction to stay with their own class; every venue was a mix of ages, talents and sobriety as the campus rocked. The final night was capped by a huge fireworks/music show, followed the next morning by the famous P-rade in which alumni from all classes marched around campus and into the stadium. Even our two miniature dachshunds sported Princeton dog collars in the P-rade.

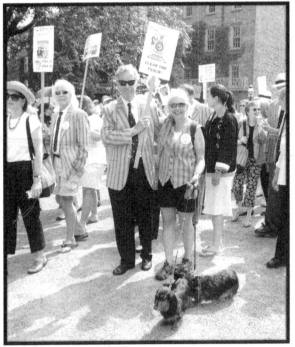

Princeton P-rade with Jester and Addie

At Reunions people asked questions, conversations ensued, and new relationships were formed. I was always treated as if I attended the university, even though women were not allowed in those olden days (as if I could have gotten in). In 2007 I made friends with one of Doug's classmates, Harry Williams, one of many thoughtful people who changed my life. Months after I was diagnosed with Parkinson's, Harry saw a piece on TV about neuroscientist Dr. Jay Alberts and his work with cycling and Parkinson's and sent us the link. Much more on that later.

While we were suffocating in a fourth-floor dorm room (with the bathroom in the basement), our daughter called to say she was engaged. Since she and her dad share a birthday, the day she called, May 31, was his sixty-second and her thirty-second birthday. The wedding that would be in September became the focal point for many of our conversations as we rolled from place to place.

Doug had arranged for us to spend a day shortly after Reunions at Gettysburg with Professor James McPherson, author of many insightful Civil War books including Pulitzer Prize winner: *The Battle Cry of Freedom*, arguably the best one-volume treatment of the Civil War. Professor McPherson invited us to join a bicycle tour of Gettysburg he was leading for the board of the Gettysburg Foundation. As we typically do, we stood at the front of the group at nearly every stop, asking multitudes of questions. Professor McPherson would either love us or hate us. At the end of the day, during which we had bicycled the first day of the battle, Professor McPherson asked if we would like to attend the Foundation dinner at the Gettysburg Hotel. We raced to our RV park, showered, and did our best to look as if we belonged at a formal event. Professor McPherson invited us to sit at the table with him, his wife and honored guests. During dinner when I asked him what he liked most about giving bicycle tours of Gettysburg, his answer surprised me: "I like biking. I've heard all the questions a thousand times."

Jim apologized for having board commitments the next afternoon, but wondered if we would like to join him for at least another half day on the bikes, just the three of us. After a memorable morning, he followed us back to our van and autographed all seven of his books we had carried with us.

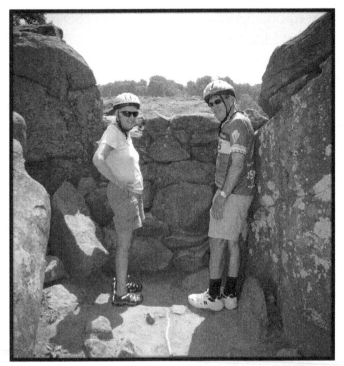

At Gettysburg's Devil's Den with Professor McPherson
(Photo by Doug Little)

With travel, Reunions, Professor McPherson and wedding plans, I never noticed I was shaking, or at least I recorded nothing about it in my journal. This corresponds with what I've heard from other PwPs who report they often don't have a sense of even having the disease when fully engaged in other activities. That engagement in the moment kept me from being aware something was amiss.

.ℓ. .ℓ. .ℓ. .ℓ. .ℓ.

Between May 31 and September 22, I experienced a few strange events that were, in retrospect, significant markers. The annual Seafair summer festival in Seattle culminated with hydroplane races and a fabulous air show. To train for an upcoming cycling adventure around Crater Lake, on August 5 Doug and I rode our bikes around half of Lake Washington, across the Mercer Island bridge and on to a party, over thirty-eight miles. After the usual revelry and a couple of beers we started to ride the additional seven miles home through traffic. For several months I had been having intermittent chest pains—a tightening in the middle followed by pains that felt like small electric shocks shooting down the length of my arms—always when I was doing some cardiovascular exercise. On the way back from the party though, my arms ached from my armpits down to my elbows, which I naively attributed to the busy day. Suddenly, without warning, a massive electrical shock painfully coursed through my left shoulder and arm, frightening us both. We stopped to see if there would be another event or if I could ride home. I rode home.

I felt fine, but fearing I had had a heart attack, I spent the next morning at the hospital going through a full battery of tests only to confirm I had the heart of a thirty-year-old. Since everything tested better than normal, I was given clearance to ride around Crater Lake the next week. The doctor assured me that rapid heartbeats are not unusual unless accompanied by lightheadedness or dizziness. Whatever happened on Seafair Sunday remains a mystery. In retrospect, my weeks of training for the ride around Crater Lake had likely mitigated my Parkinson's symptoms.

The following Sunday we loaded our van with four bikes, too much gear, four adults and two miniature dachshunds for the drive to Oregon. One person would drive while the other three cycled, taking turns at the wheel on the route to Crater Lake, the ride around the lake, and back to Seattle. When it was my turn to pedal, I had to work as hard as I could to keep up with the two men. I biked hour after hour, not realizing this cycling had anything to do with healing my shaking self.

The research from Dr. Alberts, which I later discovered, showed that benefits from forced-pace cycling generally last for four weeks with some tapering off, and another few weeks subsequent to stopping. In stark contrast, pharmacological benefits last a few hours at most. I was definitely forcing the pace of my cycling!

.♪ ♪ ♪ ♪ ♪

Since the Crater Lake ride ended five weeks before the wedding, once home, my days were filled with sewing brightly colored tablecloths and burying a queen-sized bed in huge brilliant tissue paper dahlias to use for decorating the marina for the reception. Neighbors opened their homes for our family members enabling everyone to pitch in, making the wedding preparations as much fun as the wedding.

With many balls in the air, we celebrated the rehearsal dinner for 60 people at our house, creating ethnic foods that reflected the histories of both the bride and groom before sharing the story of each dish with the guests when the party began. Since our son's name is Jason and our new son-in-law is also Jason, Doug rechristened the new Jason "Armando" and gave a wonderful introduction of Armando to the family and to himself, as he had no knowledge he was going to receive an alter (altar?) ego.

My tremor is called a "resting tremor", which means that it is only evident when my hands are still. With all the activity, my hand had no time to waste with resting. I recall it shaking somewhat at the actual wedding, which I attributed to nerves and a chill in the air, but not so much prior to that. Although I was oblivious, photos show my right fist curled in a claw position. In retrospect, once again focusing on something other than myself left no time or energy for anything else.

After the wedding, having executed all our responsibilities, we quietly drove to Yellowstone in our little camper van to relax. With no more biking, just fishing, I became increasingly aware of my hand shaking on the steering wheel. I sat on it (the hand) or placed it low on the wheel or between my legs hoping Doug might not notice. I rubbed my forearm in unsuccessful efforts to take away the ache. I ignored it. As I became more and more affected by this strange body part, I couldn't deny the increasing shaking, general weakness and sense of confusion I felt. I couldn't hide my brain under my hamstrings. Still, despite mounting evidence of significant changes in my body, I denied that anything might be systemically amiss.

Chapter 3. Puzzle Pieces

Casting soft-hackle flies quarter-down to spawning trout in the Madison River in Yellowstone—an excellent time to contemplate reality, a hard time to sustain denial.

We fly-fish a lot, especially in the fall in Yellowstone country, when deeply colored spawning trout fill the rivers. Bugling elk, howling coyotes and eerie cries of sandhill cranes add surreal magic to the landscape. One of my favorite haunts is the bend on the Madison River eleven miles from the West Yellowstone entrance to Yellowstone National Park, known locally as Eleven Mile.

Each time I wade into the weedy, cold, rushing water, casting soft hackles and streamers on long lines, sweeping the banks where hefty fish inevitably hang out, I'm acutely aware that maintaining my balance while wading deep weed beds in strong currents is always an issue. I recall no difficulties with my balance that fall. Just with other things.

That late September I stood at Eleven Mile casting my Christmas soft hackle to spawning rainbows and browns. I remember the fly because I created it: Nan's Christmas Soft Hackle, a silver hook covered with green peacock hurl, ribbed with red wire, secured with a red head. Red and green: a gift.

A big rainbow trout snatched the fly, spurted to fast water and weed beds, shaking its head to try to rid itself of the pain in its lip. Instead of reeling smoothly, my hand jerked, and jerked again. My arm got so tired I braced the butt of the rod against my stomach and struggled to get the fish to the net. When I finally did net it, I struggled to extract the fly. It was a good-sized fish, maybe 19 inches. I rested after all that effort, puzzled. Hoping that this was an anomaly, I cast again only to have it happen again.

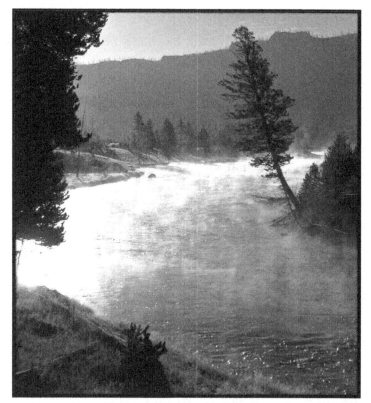

Morning mist at Eleven Mile on the Madison in Yellowstone
(Photo by Doug Little)

Through the fall trip I struggled to land fish, even smaller ones. Whereas it used to take just a couple of minutes, in 2007 I took five to eight minutes to get fish to the net and several tries to actually net them before awkwardly and painfully removing flies with almost no strength in my right hand. I stood, exhausted, frustrated and upset at my painfully inadequate efforts. For years I have always thanked the fish as I slid them back into the current. That fall I added an apology to each of these beautiful creatures and did my best to make sure they were ready before letting them swim off. I worried that some fish may have died.

I tried to blow off my strange inadequacies like most people do when they notice something amiss but don't want to acknowledge an uncomfortable reality—until the day my fishing problem went public. At Barns Hole Number Two on the Madison I caught a 21-inch rainbow and had to back up to the shore to land it. People crowded around, but as I tried and tried to get the fly out, my fingers refused to work. I reached for my hemostat as someone volunteered, "You're killing the fish! Let me do it." I didn't answer. As I finally extracted the fly and carefully released the fish, I felt horrible, incredibly old and inadequate. I stopped fishing the Barns.

ƨ ƨ ƨ ƨ ƨ

Physical problems were one thing, but mental problems posed even more inexplicable challenges. One night at the Madison campground I felt so strange, my brain not fully functioning. I couldn't recall where the dog leashes were stored, the same place they had been stored all along. I had difficulty sequencing what we had done over the last several days. In my journal I considered, "Maybe I am losing my mind. Doug just took the dishes to wash in the cold-water sink. I think we have been heating water here in the van to wash up, and he says no, we've been washing in cold water. My brain feels very strange; I don't know what it is real and what is not. He took the dishes and left."

We stayed in the Yellowstone area for nearly six weeks, driving our van from river to river, enjoying the lack of pressure, crowds, changing weather, bugling elk, dustings of snow and many fish on our lines. Whenever my arm wasn't busy it shook unless I was sitting on my hand. I adapted to problems with the reel and releasing fish, thinking of this as a temporary "new normal." A few times I cried while trying to tie on small flies with unstable fingers. That fall I lost more flies due to bad knots than I had in all the years I'd been fishing.

Then, home to the whirl of the holidays. The activities of November and December exacerbated the shaking hand, various cognition errors, bumping into walls, tripping on my shoes and extreme weariness. I ignored my abnormalities.

Doug's group of buddies, The Torrs, celebrated the holidays with a fun run/scavenger hunt, sort of a silly Amazing Race around Seattle. Traditionally the spouses kept time and ensured that the nonsensical rules were followed. In 2007 the women were allowed to participate in the actual "race". Dorothy and LuAnn, both at least four years my senior, and I comprised a team. LuAnn had flown in from Europe the night before, returning from winning her age group in the international Concept II rowing finals. Even though there weren't many competitors in the her age category, her achievement was notable. Most obvious to all of us was the fact that I couldn't keep up. Finally Dorothy carried my light backpack, leading the way from location to location. By the time I arrived, they had found the next clue. I generally deciphered it and we were off to find the next one, Dorothy and LuAnn leading, me lagging. LuAnn cheered me on. (Despite my less than stellar performance, we won the event.) I added the experience to my growing, unmentionable list of inexplicable failings.

♪ ♪ ♪ ♪ ♪

The year 2008 started on an excruciatingly painful wrong foot with the death of a former colleague from the University of Washington. An elder of the Muckleshoot Tribe, Willard Bill, Sr. had taught a class called "Educating Native Americans" at the UW for many years. I had been a guest speaker in his class, not because I'm Native American, since I'm not, but because as an anthropologist I had worked closely with tribes to build programs for Native high school students to prepare them to be successful in science and math at the college level. Willard was buried January 2, 2008.

Willard had two funerals, one on the Muckleshoot Tribe reservation and the other in a church near my home. As I parked in front of the church, I saw, but didn't see, a fire hydrant right next to the car. Nothing in my head screamed, "Don't park here!" During the service when we stood to sing, my hand shook so hard I nearly threw the hymnal into the head of the person in front of me. Dizzy, out of place, worried about the two-hour parking limit, sad about Willard and unable to process what was going on in any coherent manner, I wondered if I were losing my mind.

When I left the church I was actually surprised to see no car, just an empty space where it had been. What was going on in my brain? By this time, unaware both that I had Parkinson's and the positive effect cycling had on the disease, I had not ridden my bike since the prior August. All my riding benefit to that point had been purely fortuitous coincidence.

As I stared at the vacant space next to the hydrant, I felt like I was in a vortex of events not happening to me. Still overcome with confusion and having no conscious awareness that anything was wrong with me, I attributed my behaviors to Willard's funeral. Apparently I functioned quite well for someone who was losing her mind.

Doug drove me to the impoundment lot. (One wonders how they expect people to get from where they left their vehicle to the lot miles away.) It's hard to recall that night, except to say I felt as though I'd had an out-of-body experience. I went through the motions, paid a huge amount of money, and drove home. I don't recall Doug making any disparaging remarks. I don't know why not. I certainly deserved them.

Chapter 4. Puzzle Pieces Fit Together: Scary Picture

Some people experience extreme good fortune. I'm one of them. (This must be one of the lemonade parts of the story.) At a neighborhood holiday party in December 2007 I met a neighbor, Micki Lippe, a well-known jewelry designer. I know nothing about jewelry and had never heard of her. She never held it against me. She invited me to try out her hiking group to see if they approved of me and I thought I might like to spend a

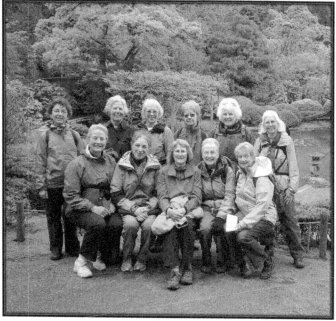

DAWGS hiking group

day each week with them. I've been with the DAWGs (Day Away Women's Group) ever since. Rules: No men, no dogs, no kids. Hike, cross-country ski or snowshoe every Thursday except holidays. Party. Love each other. Everyone should have such a great group.

One of the DAWGs was married to a doctor, which meant the other women felt free to ask her for medical advice. On Valentine's Day, on the way back from a great day of skiing, I asked Fernne if she had any thoughts about my shaking hand or why I was so weary. She dryly noted she was not the doctor in the family and her recommendation would be for me to see my doctor and ask the same questions. The elephant sat squarely on the table.

This was different from Doug's observations about my shaking hand. When we sat on the couch doing crosswords together in the mornings, he would tell me to stop shaking because it was annoying. "Why don't you sit on it or something?" For him, my hand fit in the annoying but treatable bad breath category.

Spurred by Fernne's comment, the next week I saw my doctor. She told me I had Parkinsonian symptoms but she didn't think I had Parkinson's. For a definitive diagnosis though, she recommended I see Dr. John Roberts, a movement disorder specialist (Parkinson's doctor). The earliest opening he had was March 13, nearly a month away. Not good enough. I'm not a patient person.

As soon as I walked in the door at home I called our friend Laird, a retired movement disorder specialist who used to work with Dr. Roberts. Since she couldn't come over until the next day, I sat at the computer learning everything I could about Parkinson's and Parkinsonian variations on the theme. Nothing looked promising.

When Laird came over the next day, February 22, she followed me into the house, did a few simple tests and gently told me I have Parkinson's. I thought—hoped—she was kidding. Her comment was just so final, unchallengeable. I challenged her. "What! How can you tell so quickly? Don't you need me to perform some parlor tricks or anything?" Then, sadder, "What does this mean for my life?"

We did the parlor tricks, the standard series of movement tests called the Unified Parkinson's Disease Rating Scale (UPDRS) used to assess Parkinson's patients: no blood draw, no urine sample, no brain scan, no empirical evidence; she just recorded points in the circle after each question on the UPDRS test. Even I could tell easily how badly I failed every test. She told me she could pick out a person with Parkinson's across a football field. I believe her, partly because now I can identify many of us too. Not realizing it had just changed dramatically, I thought my life was finished.

Parkinson's disease: a chronic degenerative neurological disorder affecting both body and mind. "Spirit" should be added to the definition. Laird sat with me for an hour while I whimpered and tried to hear what she was saying. She told me I have a light case of PD. Parkinson's Lite. I would rather have Miller Lite. I should expect very few changes for the next five years, she said. The average age of adult onset Parkinson's is sixty-two years and four months. I was sixty-two years and four months. By age sixty-seven I should expect an accelerating slide down the slippery slope. Lots to absorb.

🎗 🎗 🎗 🎗 🎗

By the time these symptoms, my symptoms, appeared, up to 70–80 percent of a part of my brain, the substantia nigra, had died. Was dead. Dead. She told me part of my brain was dead. That's a horrific thing to hear and try to absorb. The dead part controls fluidity of movement and provides joy juice. The dying had been going on for years but my brain had been compensating until it was finally overwhelmed. People with Parkinson's have a hard time laughing or even smiling. The happy factor is missing. So is our sense of smell, which can be a bonus at times. We typically develop a "Parkinson's mask," a non-expressive face showing little or no affect. In an article in *The New Yorker,* Michael Kinsley referred to the look as "professorial" until people realized it was "Parkinsonian." Then it wasn't professorial anymore, just scary.

In Parkinson's a primary division exists between those with tremors and those who do not shake. Apparently most tremor-dominant PwPs progress more slowly along the disease spectrum. Laird said my version is tremor dominant, hence the tag "PD Lite". The key word "apparently" refers to the designer element of the definition: nothing is certain about individual expression or progression of the disease. The only certainty at this point is that PD is incurable, in spite of claims made by wishful thinkers.

PwPs often suffer from a loss of *balance*, which makes us appear to be drunk, therefore bringing up a whole other set of social and physical issues, such as whether or not you are allowed to board an airplane. Once PwPs fall and break our bones, we start down another path, where full recovery seems unlikely. We suffer from *bradykinesia*, or slowness of movement, so that going anywhere with us is a challenge for people who move at a normal pace. Sometimes we not only move slowly, we don't even move at all. This is called *freezing*. After using the primary drug for Parkinson's, levodopa, over several years in increasing doses, many people develop *dyskinesias*, the jerky movements that make us spill soup all over our shirts. We may develop *dystonia*, uncontrolled cramping or pulling of the muscles in random directions, such as my hand curled in a claw at Jodie's wedding. Because one arm stops swinging when we walk, *rigidity* is one of the critical identifying factors for Parkinson's.

Not surprisingly, over half of PwPs suffer from depression. Of greater concern to me is the fact that up to 80 percent of us develop dementia—not Alzheimer's but a relative, I'm told: Lewy body dementia. Dementia nonetheless. Dementia scares me the most. I like thinking and remembering and enjoying life. In many respects, our stories define who we are. If we lose our stories, do we lose ourselves?

Those are big, broad categories of problems, but they only scratch the surface. *Constipation* and/or its opposite are both painful and embarrassing to live with. You want gas? We've got gas. Joint pain? Sometimes it feels like you'd like to cut off the offending member. You look at other people holding a pen, easily writing their names or taking notes and you recall when you could do that too. But because of *micrographia*, extremely tiny writing, you can no longer sign your name or read anything you pretend to write. Oddly enough you keep on trying, as if at some magical moment you will be able to read your writing again. You keep a pen in your purse. You tell your body part to do something, and it does something else. Perhaps, like me, you can no longer brush your teeth. I learned about all those unhappy variations on the theme, but did not experience most of them until later on. Lots to look forward to.

♪ ♪ ♪ ♪ ♪

So far, only Laird and I knew. She spent an hour trying to comfort me while telling me candidly (I deal better with truth than lies) what was happening and what to expect. Immediately after, I recalled almost none of the good stuff and most of the bad stuff. Doug arrived home, and we spent another hour going through what all this meant. Doug asked questions, getting a much clearer picture of the disease, its possible/probable progression and how I could help myself and receive help. Laird emphasized that, above all, I was not to go to the Internet and look up articles and interviews of people with Parkinson's. Most of them were out of date and many were just nonsense. The best thing I could do for myself was to exercise and keep active mentally as well as physically. As soon as Laird left, I raced straight to the computer, read the banned articles and watched Oprah awkwardly interview Michael J. Fox. I wept until my heart nearly broke. Doug tried to help. I don't recall what he said, other than emphasizing "Parkinson's

Lite . . . not an extreme case by any means . . . five years before I would notice any big differences." He reminded me that Laird had said because I have Parkinson's Lite I should not expect to be like Michael J. Fox in the near future. To be like him in any future scared me. Rather than being comforted, I just didn't believe him.

۔ ۔ ۔ ۔ ۔

Once I had Laird's preliminary diagnosis, the experiences of the prior months made sense. This was no slow, glacial progression of the disease. I had clearly noticed many changes in myself well before I was officially diagnosed. What would five years, fifteen years, bring? Where was my life going? I read and watched for hours, becoming more upset with each website.

Sometimes I feel like I live in a world where all the people are crazy, but because we all are, everyone pretends we're not. How crazy is it to go visit a total stranger who watches you walk up and down a hallway, tap your toes and heels, touch your finger to his finger and your nose, etc., then listen to this stranger tell you your brain is on its way out and your self-definition has changed from Person to Person with Parkinson's? You learn you will stuff yourself with pills for the rest of your life. You won't get better.

I say this because when I was diagnosed with Parkinson's, Laird told me it was because of the way I walked, the way I didn't swing my arm and the way my hand was clenched. Dr. Roberts said the same thing when I met him a month later. No empirical test. No such thing was available then, and not much is available now. They can't biopsy the brain until it is past time for fixing the disease.

Potential PwPs rely on doctors to observe our movements and tell us what disease we have. Lots of things mimic Parkinson's symptoms, too many to even begin to describe. I've met people who jerk, have tremors, lose their balance or live with all manner of symptoms, but they don't have Parkinson's. Some people go from doctor to doctor, diagnosis to diagnosis, drug to drug, following no clear roadmap. One of my friends took the wrong medication for fifteen years in increasing doses, until he learned he didn't actually have Parkinson's: his symptoms represented side effects from his medications, not from his problem. When he tried bicycling and got no relief, he sought a second opinion. Once he got off the high doses of multiple medications, he said his legs hadn't felt so strong since I knew him in high school.

Diagnosis, February 22, 2008, was a difficult day.

🐾 🐾 🐾 🐾 🐾

The day after my diagnosis we headed up to Whistler, British Columbia, for a few days of skiing. Driving north to the Canadian border, we were unusually quiet as we thought about coming changes and how we would cope. Doug and I do a lot of things together, often outside and somewhat challenging. We ski, hike, fish, garden, bike and just generally have a good time out-of-doors. We also travel a lot, exploring unusual places. How was Parkinson's going to impact our relationship? It certainly would make an impact. Things would change. Although we were in our sixties, it had not really occurred to us to talk much about end-of-life decisions or what we would do if . . . Now my brain was working overtime.

Although when we had visited Whistler only a month earlier I had skied just fine, all of a sudden I feared it would be very difficult, perhaps impossible, for me to ski. The needle on my anxiety meter registered ten. Doug assured me not a whole lot had changed in the last few weeks. We just had different knowledge now, and we would adjust as we learned how this was going to play out. I felt so sad; perhaps this would be my last season skiing. Clearly I overreacted, but I couldn't help myself.   The anxiety associated with Parkinson's was real beyond expression.

As we drove north and I tried to come to grips with this new reality, oddly enough I couldn't recall either the name of my disease or the description of it as "chronic degenerative." I drove along, thinking, "I have . . . what is it I have? What letter does it start with? I can't ask Doug the name of my disease. Figure it out." Finally, after some thought, Aha! Parkinson's disease. How will I remember it? I need a clue. Yellowstone Park. If I can think of Yellowstone Park, I'll surely recall the name of my disease. *Park*inson's disease, a . . . what kind of disorder?   Two words describe it.   Two words.   Chronic, chronic, chronic.   What will trigger *chronic* in my mind? Kronos Quartet. Yellowstone Park, Kronos Quartet. The other word? Degenerative. Degenerative. Degenerative. Not easy to find a word clue for degenerative. Ellen DeGeneres. Why her? Why not? Yellowstone Park plus Kronos Quartet plus Ellen DeGeneres equals my disease."

I recognized later I was going through emotional shock. My brain, heart and spirit had shut down enough to give me space and time to absorb the unthinkable, unacceptable truth facing me: I had Parkinson's disease. Some people shut down and don't come back from an emotional shock like this. I felt overwhelmed, terrified of not coming back.

I also realized much later that I had chosen happy things as my mnemonic clues. It was a curious juxtaposition of happy and sad, not intentional, all subconscious.   But my clues worked. Sometimes I had to wait for them, but in the ensuing weeks, when I was often at a loss to name the disease, Yellowstone, Kronos and Ellen never let me down.

Neither did Doug and our kids and their spouses. When we told our kids, they responded predictably.   Jason and Christy, our son and daughter-in-law, asked a million questions and shared their confidence in me and their love. Jodie and Jason, our daughter and son-in-law (apparently all boys born in a certain five-year period were named Jason), came over with flowers, questions and hugs. Right from the outset I experienced the beginning of what would be an anchor for my wellness: a depth of loving care from important people in my life, especially family. (More lemonade!)

Once I sorted out Yellowstone, The Kronos Quartet and Ellen, my mind began to dwell on the inevitable, inexorable course of the disease. I pictured myself shaking violently, so scaring small children that I would avoid public contact, slurring my words—an unintelligible, wheelchair-bound bobblehead—drooling, not a wife, mother or grandmother. Terrifying images.

My neighbor, heart surgeon Dr. Lester Sauvage, has Parkinson's and when he held my hands and told me I would be fine, I believed him. He said we were comrades and I believed that too. I knew that someday I would hope to be able to look in someone's eyes like Lester had looked into mine and convince them they have what it takes to live a full life with this disease. The challenge ahead was defining what it meant to live a full life. There must be more to my existence than inspiring others.

Doug and I had retired early, anticipating at least ten to fifteen years of good health to enjoy each other, our life and the world. But there we were, like my brother Tom says, ducks being shot at in a carnival booth, traveling round and round, never knowing when or how we're going to get hit, or if we'll just keep going round and round. I was the first duck hit in our family, even though I'm the youngest of four siblings.

Still gripping the wheel as we drove north, I began making heavy pronouncements. I promised to keep my independence as long as possible. If I asked for help, it meant I needed it. Doug should not question anything I asked, but just do it. I've been known to milk situations now and then, but I blithely promised it would not happen again. (With some notable slippages, I'm keeping the pledge.)

As though I had one foot in the grave, I offered sacrifices. Having observed that many nursing homes rely on spouses to be daily caregivers for loved ones suffering with diseases such as Parkinson's, one person giving up their life for the other, I did not want that role for Doug and I suspected he didn't want it either. I told him that as far as I know we have only one life to live and I was concerned about what impacts this disease would have on his life. I righteously announced that he shouldn't miss out just because my brain went on holiday. "So," I solemnly told him, "when the time comes, I don't want you to hesitate to put me in a home so you can keep on with your life." He looked at me with a straight face and answered, oh so sincerely, "I've been thinking about that and I've decided to advertise for another partner on Craigslist." We laughed and realized another hurdle was behind us. I cried a little too. I can't imagine going through this alone.

When our kids were little we put them in the Alpental Ski School at nearby Snoqualmie Pass. One thing led to another over the years until all four of us ended up as instructors. I'm an intermediate skier, but I enjoy the challenge of making my way down most slopes. I recall all too clearly my lack of coordination when I got off the first lift at Whistler, post-diagnosis. I skied like a beginner, thinking through every weight shift, avoiding moguls, falling more than I had in years. By the second day I was skiing normally again. Shocking to note, the world hadn't ended after all.

I had no trouble remembering I had a disease. Like a loud clanging in my ears, reminding me to face reality, not to pretend everything was just like it was before, it was all I could think about. Everything was not as it was before. This was the beginning of the end of my life as I knew it. What made me think I could ski or do anything I used to do before? Fool.

I still feel sick to my stomach when I think about those days when I made my transition from a *Person* to a *Person with Parkinson's*. I also feel tremendous empathy for those who have just been diagnosed and for their families and loved ones. Even in the month before we saw Dr. Roberts, we both noted the disease was getting old very quickly. Doug asked about my day and got annoyed when I told him how hard it was to focus. "You're just blaming everything on this," he growled. I realized it might take a long time for us both to adjust.

An old friend, who has had more than her share of difficulties in life, called to console me: "I'm not going to tell you everything is going to be all right; I am going to tell you that Nan Little has grit." That helped.

Rather late in life I earned a doctorate in anthropology with a focus on trying to understand how Native Americans best learn science and mathematics. After years of study and a multitude of experiences in conferences, in conversations and being with Indian people, I concluded that the core element of Native American instruction is storytelling. A person makes a point by telling a story. Rather than telling the audience what they are supposed to understand from hearing the story, they trust each listener to take away whatever is important to them at that time. At first the understanding may be rather superficial, but as the story is told and retold it gains depth of meaning. Each time the storyteller tells it or the listener hears it, the story is slightly different because both listener and narrator are a little bit different. As everyone hears multiple iterations, they keep redefining what is important until it becomes an intrinsic part of them. Indians are fabulous storytellers.

I'm finding the same thing applies to Parkinson's. At first I could hear, from Laird and then Dr. Roberts and the Internet and a few other people who have Parkinson's, what it is like to have the disease. But as I experienced the story over and over again from multiple points of view, both personally and from others, I began to understand in depth what it means to have Parkinson's. I continue to learn. Even though I suffered emotional shock when I heard the diagnosis, the essential me eventually reemerged. Parkinson's stories are my stories.

♪ ♪ ♪ ♪ ♪

A basic test to confirm a Parkinson's diagnosis is to observe the patient's response to carbidopa/levodopa (C/L), called Sinemet: those PwPs who respond to the drug probably have the disease. If they don't respond, they may be given a higher dose of C/L, or other drugs, or a combination of drugs. In that Oprah interview with Michael J. Fox he told her he had taken a whole bathtub full of drugs in order to be able to make it through the show. Maybe he exaggerated a little, not a whole bathtub, but probably a whole handful.

Diagnosing Parkinson's reminds me of a dart game: some doctors have better aim than others. Instead of giving me the gold-standard C/L when I was diagnosed, Dr. Roberts gave me a dopamine agonist, a 2 mg Neupro patch to wear. It was great! Dopamine agonists frequently are prescribed as the first drug, especially for young PwPs, when symptoms do not warrant the more powerful Sinemet. As soon as I started the patch some symptoms disappeared, or at least were mitigated. The tremor was still there, but I was a bundle of energy and happier than I had been in months. I didn't even need a nap during the day. With such a small dose, all I probably experienced was a placebo effect. But I didn't care. It worked! One week after I was put on Neupro it was pulled from the market and didn't reappear again for several years. Naturally I was given another dopamine agonist, hoping it would have the same effect. So much for hope.

I don't know why, but I expected any medicine I took after Neupro would fail. Possibly the power of my fear doomed the medicine. Dr. Roberts told me Mirapex should work equally well and I should not have any serious side effects other than constipation, nausea, excessive sleepiness and a few other treasures. I should be aware, however, that one reaction to Mirapex might be obsessive behavior. Obsessive behavior. If he only knew!

I went to hell in a handbasket, but I didn't know if it was the medication or the disease. (A constant conundrum: Which is worse, the symptoms or the side effects of the medication?) "Hell in a handbasket." What does that mean? Although difficult to deal with, the physical symptoms were nothing compared to my mental problems.

I suffered from hallucinations: he was stark naked, young, and very handsome. Astonished beyond belief, I rolled up onto my elbow to get a better look. He wasn't there. Lying next to me was my threescore-plus husband clad in his pajamas, under the covers. Oh well. The next week two young men appeared silhouetted against the window in our bedroom. Although they visited on different nights, their demeanor was remarkably similar. I knew they weren't there because the dogs didn't bark. If it weren't for the dogs, I would have sworn they were real, but each time I blinked and lifted my head, they disappeared. Once when I was driving on the freeway a huge truck in the lane next to me prevented me from merging. I looked forward, and then glanced again to the right. No truck. Hallucinations were only part of it.

Obsessive behavior consumed my days and nights. Although never much interested in needlework, I picked up cross-stitch with a passion, making cross-stitch pictures of national parks, bouquets of flowers, scriptures, marching penguins, Christmas ornaments—I couldn't stop. On our fishing trips, often I would wake up at two thirty or three o'clock in the morning and stitch for hours inside my sleeping bag with a flashlight in my teeth. Finally I could sleep for a couple of hours before I would be up and at it again. In a little over a month I stitched two large pictures of Yellowstone, more than one hundred thousand stitches each, along with numerous works that cover every panel in the van. All relatives have cross-stitch mementoes of this phase of my life. It's a wonder I didn't go blind or lose the use of my fingers. We have a lot of pretty artwork, but the cost was tremendous, no sleep night after night.

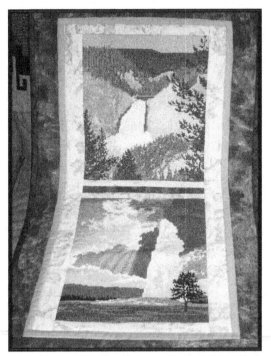

Cross-stitch of Yellowstone, 240,000 stitches

When my friend, Carol, from West Yellowstone, taught me how, I began quilting with a vengeance. If I weren't cross-stitching by hand, I was focused at the sewing machine quilting as though each quilt had a deadline. And each one had to be just right. I magnified pictures to figure out the mathematics to transform a quilted wall hanging into a bedspread. Pretty tricky. I've never been good with numbers and now, with medication and PD, I could barely do math at all, much less transpose hundreds of tiny little pieces correctly to make a queen-sized quilt. But I did it. I doubt if anyone but my teacher would find the one mistake.

At one point I had a panic attack, my first. On a fishing trip I thought I was lost, even though there were signs and landmarks all around telling me where I was. I could read but not comprehend, not even a simple map right in front of my face. I was terrified I wouldn't return to the van in time to take my medicine, forgetting I had my medicine in my fishing vest. I started to cry and to babble, puzzling two nearby fishermen. Since they knew where our van was, one of them told me to get in his car and he drove me to it, no more than a quarter of a mile away on a road with no turns. I felt like a fool. I was a fool. The medicine made me a fool, not my own self. I knew I was losing my mind.

I became both illiterate and inarticulate. Formerly an avid reader, I could no longer read. I could decode words, but without a sense of content I did not know what I had read or who wrote it. Social gatherings were a bust. If more than one conversation was going on, I could not follow either, much less add any intelligent commentary. At parties I stood stupidly while my friends shared information, ideas and plans. It was all I could do to keep from crying. I didn't want to go anywhere. I didn't want to meet anyone. I wanted to hide. I hid by being quiet.

I endured one horrible experience after another, realizing this must be what it's like to go mad. While you're going mad, you know what's happening. Once you've gone mad, it doesn't matter anymore except to your family and those who love you. The transition is the killer.

After suffering with Mirapex for months, my husband and I spoke to Dr. Roberts to see if I could take a different medicine. We switched to another dopamine agonist equal to the Mirapex dosage: 8 mg of Requip XL. Although the major horrors were gone, it seemed as if I could do better with less medicine, so we cut it back to 6 mg and then a few months later, after becoming an avid high cadence cyclist, to 4 mg. I remained stabilized on the reduced regimen for several years.

Chapter 5. More Pedaling to Health

In September 2008, Harry Williams, a college classmate of Doug's, forwarded a video clip of a segment he had seen on the *NBC Nightly News* about interesting work being done by research neuroscientist Jay Alberts, Ph.D., at the Cleveland Clinic. In the video, Dr. Alberts demonstrated the positive effects of high cadence cycling on Parkinson's symptoms. Having grown up in Iowa and being a premier cyclist, he had convinced several of his friends to join him in 2003 riding across Iowa in *The Des Moines Register*'s big bike ride: the Register's Annual Great Bike Ride Across Iowa (RAGBRAI, pronounced rag-brī, rhymes with "eye"), the oldest cross-state, multiday bike ride in the nation.

One of Jay's friends had brought his wife who had Parkinson's, intending to ride tandem, but they had never ridden a tandem before. When the husband dismounted, forgetting his wife on the back, it looked like a painful, emotional week ahead for the group. To keep his friends out of divorce court, Jay volunteered to ride the "captain's" seat, the front of the bike. As Jay typically rides at 80–90 rpm, she had to also, since on a tandem the pedals are linked. By midweek, she reported she felt as if she didn't have Parkinson's any more, and by the end of the week her handwriting, which suffered from the usual Parkinson's micrographia, was nearly normal.

His interest piqued, Jay designed an experiment using ten patients at similar stages in their Parkinson's progression. Five were paired with power riders on tandem stationary bikes, cycling for three one-hour sessions each week, with a 10-minute warm-up followed by 40 minutes at the 80–90 rpm cadence and a 10-minute cool-down. After eight weeks, this group had reduced their Parkinson's UPDRS rating by 35 percent, a major improvement. The second group of five on solo stationary bikes cycled the same amount of time but at their normal cadence of about 55 rpm on average. They gained in fitness but experienced no change in their Parkinson's rating. Research is ongoing, but these initial published results were enough to be reported on the *NBC Nightly News.* Thus began our relationship with Dr. Alberts as Pedaling For Parkinson's (PFP) entered my life. This was the first time I felt encouraged since my initial reaction to the Neupro patch.

I contacted Jay and began biking on my own—sporadically through the winter cold and rain—but continued to deteriorate, with psychological as well as physical symptoms upsetting my life. In early spring Jay emailed me an article he had had published outlining these cycling protocols, emphasizing the importance of maintaining a pace of 80–90 rpm for 40 minutes three times per week, keeping my heart rate at 60-85% of Maximum Heart Rate (MHR). Appendix A summarizes these protocols.

Jay also invited us to join the PFP team in the 2009 RAGBRAI. Without thinking, I agreed, conveniently ignoring that I was sixty-three years old, a woman and I had Parkinson's. Plus, no one had ever looked at me seriously and said "athlete." However, since RAGBRAI had sat squarely on Doug's bucket list for several years, it was an easy sell to get us on board. He had links: Doug's mom and dad grew up in Iowa and graduated from Iowa State. He looked forward to seeing the land and possibly tracking down some distant relatives. He had enjoyed Cycle Montana and relished the idea of being part of *the* big ride. I didn't realize we were signing up for 450 miles of biking up and over hills and more hills and a few more hills for seven days, adding up to over 23,000 feet in elevation gain. Since one of my Parkinson's symptoms was extreme fatigue, I could only imagine how it would feel to take on RAGBRAI during the third week of July in toasty Iowa!

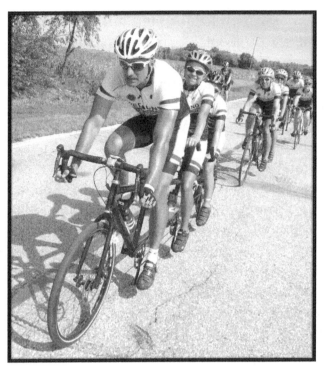

Jay Alberts with Abbie and Grant on a triple at RAGBRAI
(Photo courtesy of Leigh Atkins)

Terrified of failure, I began training in earnest at an almost laughable pace. I rode over eighteen miles at least four days each week, with one or more longer rides nearly every week, sometimes thirty to forty miles, other times fifty miles, doing my best to maintain a cadence of 80–90 rpm. We took one overnight bike trip, with eighty miles the first day and thirty-five miles the second day. After that weekend, my legs twitched so badly I couldn't sleep all night. (Who knew the paper was delivered at 3:15 a.m.?) I learned the hard way about the necessity of drinking fluids along the way and stopping to rest.

Only one long month after starting my impassioned race from failure, I had a most amazing experience. As I was walking our two miniature dachshunds, Jester and Addie, I suddenly realized my body felt very different. I looked down to see both arms swinging freely by my side. I was walking upright, not shuffling along the sidewalk. My head, which had refused to turn more than a 90-degree turning radius, was fully rotational. I looked to the left. I looked to the right. I twirled my head around without pain. I went through all the motions again and yet again. Gone were the obvious symptoms that characterized me as a PwP: arm locked stiffly at my side, right hand clenched in a claw-like fist, feet shuffling along the cement, dystonia cramps curling my fingers and toes, unable to reach across my body to put on my seatbelt, leaning forward as I walked as if the sidewalk were the only interesting thing to see. My body was back!

It dawned on me that by consistently cycling at a high cadence I might be able to live a nearly normal life. There might be an opportunity for light at the end of the tunnel instead of the unremitting darkness that faced previous generations who suffered with Parkinson's. I stood on the sidewalk clutching the leashes, crying like a baby. The dogs wagged their tails.

🐾 🐾 🐾 🐾 🐾

The next week Doug and I visited my neurologist, Dr. Roberts. After his usual examination, he said he would not be able to tell I had Parkinson's except for a minor shaking of my right hand. We were all astonished.

Looking for clues, I pored through my journals for the last few years to see if I could chronicle the onset and progression of my disease, noting changes in both physical and mental indicators, also recording my pattern of cycling. Happily, I kept a rather extensive journal and was able to roughly observe my progress (decline). I graphed the outcomes and noted a dramatic change in my symptoms directly correlated to my bike time, particularly to when I committed to the high cadence pace of 80–90 rpm. By mid-spring my mental symptoms had dropped to zero. (Jay's study had not addressed cognitive effects, which are an under recognized aspect of Parkinson's). My physical symptoms, which had reached a high of twenty-two per month in the fall of 2008, had dropped to zero in only eight months. Although my data were purely anecdotal, they were a reflection of my real experience and hopefully worth sharing.

Finally I decided I would be fine for RAGBRAI 2009—not fast, but fine.

Chapter 6. A Most Difficult Barrier

On my last training ride along Lake Washington in June of 2009, a bald eagle flew along with me for a ways, a good omen for a perfect June day. Soon after, Doug and I set out in high spirits for our great Iowa adventure with our dachshunds, Jester and Addie, and moderate anxiety on my part. Could I reasonably expect to ride my bike from the Missouri to the Mississippi? To be determined. Late in the day we found a spot at the Umtanum campground on the Yakima River, then hiked across the old bridge, through fields ablaze with wildflowers, all the way to the top of the ridge, realizing how tremendously fortunate we were. The dogs romped through the fields, bubbles of black appearing randomly among the sagebrush and wildflowers.

Later we noticed Jess was eating slowly and drooling in his food. He seemed to have a hard time lapping, and his breath smelled nasty, even to me with my compromised sense of smell. We stopped in Pendleton, Oregon, the next morning to see if a vet could take a quick look at him and, hopefully, just tell us to brush his teeth with baking soda. After a brief examination he showed us an ugly malignant melanoma blocking most of Jester's throat. RAGBRAI and Parkinson's became irrelevant as we raced back to Seattle, cuddling Jester, giving as much love as possible in a short time. Our vet waited for us, confirmed the diagnosis, took samples, and did her best to prepare us for losing Jester. Possibly, just possibly, surgery might help, but she wasn't hopeful. For two days we waited anxiously for test results.

Anxiety exacerbates Parkinson's symptoms. I was a wreck, anxious beyond control, my hand flapping wildly whenever I thought of losing Jester. I could neither think sequential thoughts nor express emotions. I felt just intolerably sad. Two things helped during that awful time: being with Doug and holding and playing with Jester, who, other than not eating or drinking much, acted his normal silly self. Hoping for a miracle, we took Jester to the surgical vet but ended by saying our goodbyes to one of the best dogs ever born. That eagle? No happy omen. Just a beautiful bird flying along Lake Washington.

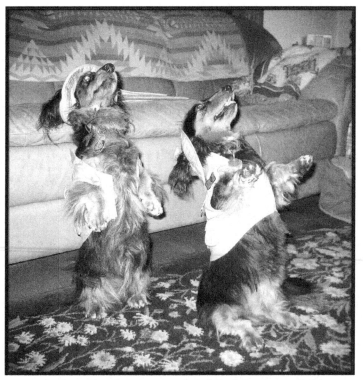

Properly attired, Jester and Addie beg to go fishing
(Photo by Doug Little)

Court Jester lived up to his name: always funny, insightful, responding to our moods, a wonderful companion. It would be hard to return to Yellowstone and Montana, to picture him playing with flopping whitefish on the shore or valiantly trying to save us from indifferent moose. Chasing a herd of cows through the tall grass with only the tip of his tail showing as he bounced like a runaway Slinky, baying all the while. Jester tolerated every small loving child who patted him with abandon, and warmed the hearts of old folks who invariably had known a dachshund when they were young.

We wondered what to do. How could we just climb in our van or get on our bikes as though nothing had happened? A metaphor for our lives, we both knew we would heal only if we moved forward and went to Iowa. Crawling into a hole was not an option. It was a long ride with many tears, as anyone who has lost a beloved dog will know.

Chapter 7. Yellowstone

To refocus physically and psychologically, we spent several days in Yellowstone cycling and fishing before driving on toward Iowa and RAGBRAI. My journal reflected my transition back to a semblance of mental health.

Late June, 2009

"On a chilly, foggy morning I ride the fourteen miles from West Yellowstone to Madison Campground. This ride calms my soul and makes me forget I have Parkinson's disease. The shoulders along the road are narrow, and in places an unfortunate four-inch drop-off could dump a cyclist into the forest or over an edge. Pinecones and little branches add hazards. Much of the ride parallels the Madison River. Aging blackened stumps, residuals of the 1989 fire, are being enveloped slowly by a new pine forest.

"On occasion I see a bald eagle across the river, perched atop one of those great black sentinels. Generally the eagle stays close to its nest on the side of the road where I'm riding. A sign admonishes drivers against stopping to gawk at the eagles. If birds are on the nest, often a nearly quarter-mile line of cars blocks the shoulder as most people ignore the sign. Cyclists can stop, and I often do. In spite of Jester, eagles fill my heart. In the spring we often see eaglets in the nest, a special thrill.

"If I am going to get over the loss of Jester, Yellowstone is the place. He is with me in my dreams and at odd moments during the days. It's calming to be on the waters, thinking about Jester some of the time, enjoying sandhill cranes, buffalo, elk, wolves, bear, coyotes, and always ravens marking the spot of a kill. Yellowstone provides ample opportunities for wonderful training rides at high elevation. We feel we are pretty much ready for RAGBRAI. Neither the loss of Jester nor Parkinson's will derail the ride."

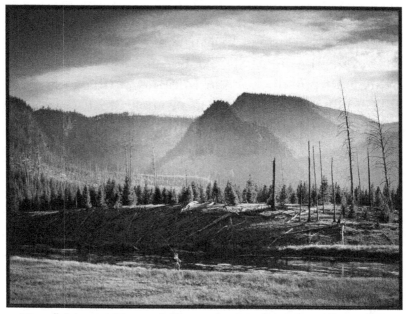

Nan fishing at Eleven Mile on the Madison in Yellowstone
(Photo courtesy of Richard Baccus)

Chapter 8. RAGBRAI Background

Naturally, when we got to Underwood, Iowa, the gathering place for the PFP group to start the 2009 ride, I was eager to meet Jay, hoping to learn more about his research and to see if I could be part of it.

I was also curious to learn about RAGBRAI, this most unlikely event. RAGBRAI: it's like Burning Man on Skinny Tires. People come from all over the world to participate. From its early beginnings as an excuse to promote small-town Iowa, it has grown from about three hundred riders to anywhere from ten to twenty thousand. For days prior to the beginning of the ride, cars stream into Iowa as though being pulled into by giant magnet. Nearly every car and bus is loaded with bicycles, gear, and jubilant cyclists. Riders come alone or in pairs or in teams, hundreds of teams, each with distinctive jerseys celebrating their creativity.

Each year Jay designs a new Pedaling For Parkinson's (PFP) jersey and bike shorts. Our first jersey with the group featured a brain with wheels and a crankshaft. Pedal the crankshaft, turn the wheels and restore some of your brain. My favorite team jerseys were worn by a group of heavyset older men whose butts sagged over their saddles. On the back of their jerseys was a dinosaur, also too big for the seat, and the proud name of the group: Team Soreassrus. Teams represented most branches of the armed services. It is my understanding they are duty bound to stop by the side of the road and help anyone in need. Whether they are duty bound or not, they certainly do help and are much appreciated.

Several traditions make RAGBRAI unique. One of my favorites is Team Roadkill. Roadkill riders each wear a ton of Mardi Gras–type bling. Whenever one of them sees the inevitable mashed possum or raccoon or squirrel or remnant of another rodent that didn't get to the other side, the riders attempt ride-by-tagging of it with their bling: beaded necklaces, cheap jewelry, anything that is shiny or bright.

Inevitably, a few riders drag along a child carrier loaded with a blaring boom box. One DJ actually broadcasts from his bike, speeding up or slowing down to interview folks along the way. Of course there are the banana bike, the guy on the unicycle, and the woman who tries to run the entire distance. Each year brings new surprises.

Since RAGBRAI is such a boon to the local economy, towns vie for months or even years to be on the route, particularly to be a stopping point. They outdo themselves with plans for activities and entertainment. One town hung a rope swing over a pond, and for five dollars one could cool off— family fun as long as riders stay clothed. This town counts on sunshine. If the masses come on a rainy or cold day, no one will care about swinging over the water. All their efforts would be wasted. As it happened, pond day 2009 was up into the nineties and the line to swing circled half the town.

It is said that RAGBRAI is the only bike ride where you gain weight. From early morning until late at night people sell treats and treasures, homemade and store-bought. During the day every church advertises yummy, homemade pie: apple, peach, cherry, banana, lemon meringue, rhubarb—any pie made by the wonderful cooks in Iowa. You want protein? Steak on a stick, pork chop on a stick, sausage on a stick. More calories? Of course: corn on a stick dipped in a vat of butter or cream-filled funnel cakes. Gatorade, water, lemonade, most things in a bottle that are nonalcoholic and portable/potable. Some water is for sale; other water is free, squirting out of hoses provided by fire departments, held up in long lines by sawhorses. While you are waiting for whatever you are waiting for, local talent, most of which is good enough to be featured on

A Prairie Home Companion, provides entertainment. Rain or shine, it's all good! Parkinson's? Forget about it!

And where do the pedaling masses sleep? None of these towns is large enough to accommodate an extra ten to fifteen thousand people in beds. Every reasonably flat square inch of grass sports a tent. Some outfitters specialize in "sagging" for RAGBRAI riders, transporting gear, precisely setting up tents in tidy rows, organizing bathroom facilities and helping their clients in whatever way is needed. Some people carry their own tents on their bikes (not very many) and some just get by.

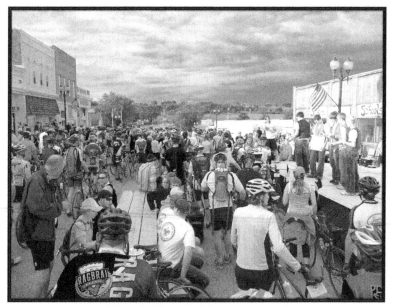

RAGBRAI entertainment (Photo by Doug Little)

Since Jay grew up in Iowa and went to school there, he has friends all over the state who know they're going to get leaned on when the ride comes anywhere near them. The PFP team has stayed with politicians, distant relatives, close relatives, in nursing homes, retirement homes and even in a funeral home. Once, faced with the prospect of no shower and no laundry facility, several of us walked across the street and approached a homeowner who was watching us pitch our tents.

We asked if we could each pay a couple of bucks to take a shower, and ten dollars for a load of laundry. Realizing we would overwhelm one house, I went next door and offered the same proposition. In no time flat we were all washed, with our clothing festively decorating branches up and down the street. Instead of just being observers, the neighbors became part of the action and had stories to tell. That's the way it is at RAGBRAI!

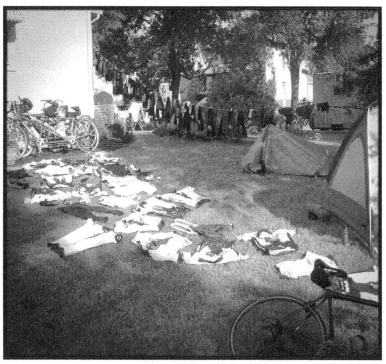

Drying our laundry at RAGBRAI
(Photo by Doug Little)

Chapter 9. RAGBRAI 2009, July 19-25

The Pedaling For Parkinson's team is still structured much as it was on the very first ride Jay took across Iowa with his friends in 2003. Most of the PFP team are friends of Jay or people who work in his lab. Few actually have the disease. This year, of the thirty-nine members of the PFP team, four of us have Parkinson's, which highlights the challenge and difficulty most people with Parkinson's have meeting such a monumental challenge as riding an average of seventy miles a day for seven days in a row. There may be more PwPs on the ride, but we four are the only ones so identified. Two are riding tandem bikes and two are on solo bikes. I have never ridden a tandem before and neither has Doug. It didn't occur to us to try.

Day 1: Fabulous!

"We just finished day one of RAGBRAI. Our group gathered 16 miles from the starting place at Council Bluffs to have a little peace the night before the ride began. (Of course the peaceful starting point added 16 miles to the first day's ride. My usual training ride is 18 miles, so I did a training ride before we even started the official trip.) The morning was cool, a few clouds overhead. After the group photo (including our dachshund, Addie), we were clipped in our pedals and rolling at 7:30.

"About 15,000 cyclists, plus or minus a few, snaked over the terrain for quite literally miles. All colors of jerseys and teams of every shape and size moved like a giant peloton over the roads. Southern Iowa is nothing but hilly.

"Our route map looked like an earthquake on a seismograph. Fly down, grind up, avoid crazy cyclists and cracks in the road. For the most part, people ride well; they are mannerly, interested in finding out who you are and why you are there. It felt like a cocktail party on wheels with no booze."

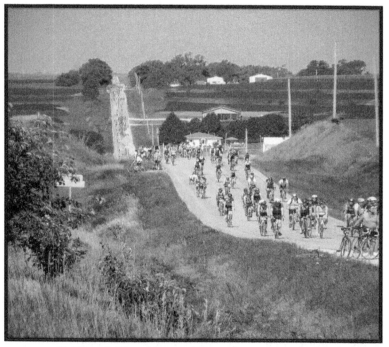

Rolling hills of Iowa (Photo by Doug Little)

"Shortly into the ride, food stands dotted the roadsides. Breakfast of every kind, sweets, water, Gatorade. Every service group, scout group, sports team, church, whatever, was out there ready to make yours a better day and theirs a fuller coffer. In addition, families parked alongside the road in lawn chairs or on little tractors and cheered us on. We drank a lot of electrolytes, ate plenty of food, and felt great.

"Tonight we're staying with a wonderful family in Red Oak who just answered a cold call asking to house

35 people overnight, plus let us use their showers and laundry. One of our guys fixed their computer. It's a beautiful evening, right out of *The Music Man*. Small-town Iowa with houses like Grandma's, big porches, hanging swings, white clapboard walls. Friendly people everywhere, all eager to welcome us. A breeze and clouds now and then."

Day 2: Still Going Strong

"Seventy-four miles with many hills, but manageable. Fortunately it was overcast and in the low 70s, perfect for riding. In the evening Jay gave a talk to a group at the Methodist Church five miles from where we were staying. Nearly all our group wanted to go, so Doug drove the van, absolutely packed, back and forth to the site. This meant driving through streams of cyclists who were still coming into Greenfield. Doug is an artist behind the wheel. I was excited to hear what Jay had to say and thrilled to be part of his team.

"This morning Jay was on Good Morning America, and tonight the local ABC affiliate interviewed him again. He asked me to join him, so I shared my story, hopefully inspiring others to follow suit. I find speaking on behalf of PFP acts as therapy for my own Parkinson's. No matter how tired I am, if anyone asks about my experience, I have a burst of energy to answer questions. I also know every TV interview includes a pan shot of my shaking hand. It has become a joke among those of us with Parkinson's."

Day 3: Adventure is Adversity Recalled

"Adventure today. We rode 79 miles with nearly a mile of elevation gain. Rain, headwinds, cross winds, cool temps and finally sun at the end of the day. I had one close call, nearly taking a header in the ditch, but fortunately avoided crashing when a fellow rode right into the tire of the man in front of me. I jumped my bike to the gravel and got my feet down to avoid pitching forward. My heart pounded crazily for a long time. I also caught my bike wheel in the cement and managed to jump my bike out of the crack rather than go head over handlebars.

"Everyone agreed it was a hard day, but everyone also agreed it was quite an adventure. The colors changed from the multi-colored jerseys of the first two days to lines of yellow and lime rain jackets. As with the days before, after the sun came out, people asked all of us PFPs about our intriguing jerseys with pictures of brains on the front and back and were truly interested in our story of cycling as a treatment for Parkinson's. In spite of being utterly worn out at the end of the day, I'm doing astonishingly well.

"At the end of the ride today (nine hours total, including time for lines for potties and food) I was so exhausted I flopped on the grass and wept for a few minutes. The men in our group stood around, not having a clue what to do with a sobbing woman. Susie, our masseuse, knew exactly what to do. Soon I recovered my composure, enjoyed a shower and had a fun evening.

"Susie Cornwall is a particularly special member of the PFP team. She joins the group each year to give massages to the people with Parkinson's and, with any time left over, to other members of the group as well. In her real life she raises horses and owns dachshunds, so she is especially well suited for driving our van and taking care of our dog during the day while Doug and I ride. Another gift from PFP!"

"Yesterday and today Jay gave talks to groups about his Parkinson's research. About 100 people attended. Tonight he asked if I would join him for the Q&A. People were so interested in seeing how his work personally affects me. I realize I am an important part of

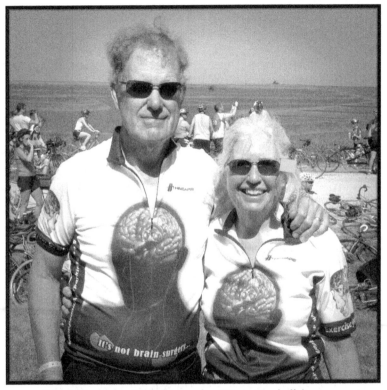

Modeling our PFP "Exercise Your Brain" jerseys

his message as well. He is a wonderful speaker with a compelling story. Although I've heard Jay speak several times, every time it's a real privilege. It's odd to think I am old enough to be his mother."

Day 4: A Truth Revealed

"We all recall the scene in *Field of Dreams* when James Earl Jones walks into the cornfield facing … what? We ponder the great question: What's next? In these four days of RAGBRAI I have discovered *the*, or at least *an*, answer. About 15,000 riders started this trek across Iowa. Most are men. Each day I see ever so many hurry into the rows of corn with looks of great expectation, anguish and pain. As they emerge they uniformly grin with relief. Women, on the other hand, wait at least a half hour in line for relief, making friends and learning each other's stories. Now that you know what's in the cornfield, watch your step!"

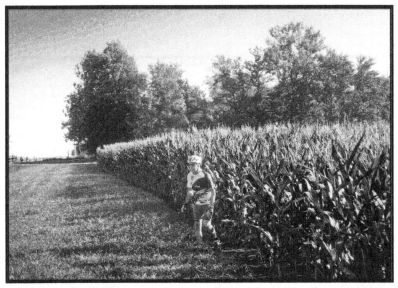

Solving the mystery of the cornfield (Photo by Doug Little)

"We started with morning low clouds casting a surreal haze over riders as we merged from our separate camping sites into increasing streams, then a river of colors once again. No wind, no rain, no need for jackets. The temperature stayed in the perfect 70s until the sun came out in late morning. By then, most of the ride was complete and we were ready to frequent, yet again, Beekman's Homemade Ice Cream trailer. Since Beekman's is homemade ice cream, they haul along the generators and the hundred-year-old equipment they use to make four flavors on the spot. Several generations of Beekman's run the stand.

"Robert Beekman has Parkinson's, and PFP helped purchase a special seat for his truck to enable him to be mobile in his community. His wife, Gloria, eagerly greets anyone from our group. Today she had me demo the seat lift as she explained how this gift completely changed their lives. It makes me even more proud to be a part of PFP. The happier I am, the less I am affected by my Parkinson's symptoms. I guess it makes sense, but this ride is giving me a tremendous infusion of energy."

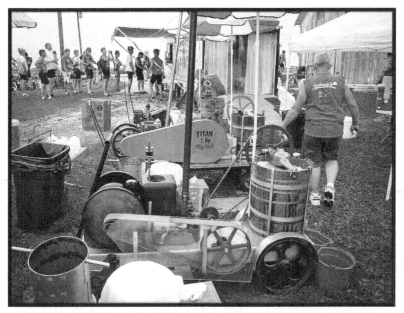

Beekman's homemade ice cream (Photo by Doug Little)

"Beekman's is just one of a number of vendors who follow the course, setting up their trucks every day. Another of the notable movable vendors, Mr. Pork Chop, has a big pink pig painted on the side of their old school bus. PB&J is always a popular stop, where you can place an order for the most unlikely things to be found in a PB&J sandwich: maybe Skittles or M&M'S, chips, pickles, or maybe even peanut butter and jelly. Rain or shine, the movable vendors are always there.

"Tonight we're staying on a farm with a little lake and animals. The children in our group are in heaven. There is a soft breeze, and thus many contented cyclists. We've checked out the TV presentations from Good Morning America and ABC5 News Des Moines. Tonight we'll grill dinner and get a good night's sleep. Tomorrow is another long day, again with hills. Today was a piece of cake (with pie and ice cream of course)."

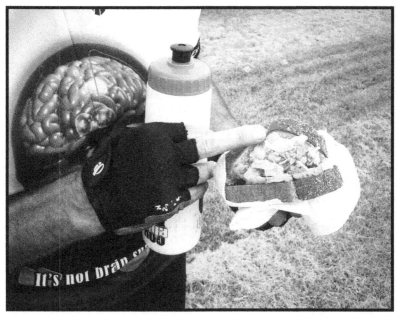

Not your everyday PB&J (Photo by Doug Little)

"This evening Jay raffled off the prizes he had collected for our team. Each year every rider is encouraged to raise funds to support the PFP program, earning one raffle ticket for each $50 we raise. Jay lays all the raffle items on the ground and places a cup next to each item. We distribute our tickets in the cups according to how badly we want a particular item. Jay's daughter selects the winning ticket from each cup. Doug and I won many jerseys and ended up trading with others. Much laughter, applause and good will."

Day 5: Weather on Our Side

"Last night we all awoke at 3:30 to horrendous rain/hail storms. It sounded like the inside of a drum in our van, but we were much better off than those in leaky tents. Needless to say, we all hit the road early. With the rain gone and weather on our side, we had a perfect day for our 75-mile ride. Some members of the group did a century (100 miles, in bike-speak), but Doug and I were more than content to just ride the planned route. A minor cloud cover kept the temperature within manageable limits. The steep hills of earlier days mellowed into tree-lined, rolling hills interspersed with corn and soybean fields. Maybe because of the rain last night, there seemed to be fewer riders today.

"I was told that in the 37 years of RAGBRAI this was the 7th hilliest route. A week ago I had no clear idea about how to ride hills. Now I knew on the downslope to put my knees together on the bar, keep my heels down, tuck my body parts in and let it rip all the way down, then up most of the next hill until I could pedal again, usually about 107 rpm, and keep it up as long as I could go, often to the top. This strategy saved me about an extra hour each day as I made my way through the 'flat' state. At first I was afraid; then I realized I loved it! The roads were perfect, allowing riders to tuck and ignore the brakes. It was so much fun! It had never occurred to me that at age 63 and with Parkinson's disease I would be swooshing downhill on a bike on a summer day in Iowa.

"We are staying out in the country near Ottumwa, at a home with a huge lawn. Our hosts were expecting five people but got 39 instead. They are fantastic. We are all well fed, showered and in clean clothes. Can't ask for more, except perhaps no thunderstorms tonight. Another 75–80 miles tomorrow, and then a 50-miler for the last day.

"It's hard to capture a single sense of this group. Everyone helps each other, cheers each other on, and laughs at each other's jokes. Although there are only four of us with Parkinson's, we feel like we are an integral part of the team. It's a wonderful group."

Day 6: The Face of Iowa

"I always thought Iowa was a flat state populated by independent-thinking folks who pretty much keep to themselves. This week proved me wrong over and over again. Although 'independent' is a good term to describe Iowans, 'keeping to themselves' is not. I doubt I have ever met such a consistently welcoming and appreciative group of people. In every town and along the route, people cheered us on. They asked where we were from and hollered their greetings of the day. Everyone gave their best efforts at giving directions, whether they knew the way or not. One woman told me she lived on the same street as our host family, but she couldn't tell me how to get there. Neither could her husband or a family friend. I ended up with three separate routes, each with several turns, and finally called Doug to see if he could guide me in.

"Day 6 registered about 80 miles on my odometer. It was cool in the morning, then hot later in the day. I came to rely on Beekman's Homemade Ice Cream as my last meal of the bike day. Most of today I felt nostalgic, sad this ride was nearly over. Oddly enough, I didn't feel tired, just contented. A very good day in a fine place."

Day 7: Final Thoughts

"Most of our group was on the road by 6:30 for the last 44 miles. I had my root beer float at 8:18 a.m.! Another beautiful day. I sang most of the way . . . 'Oh, What a Beautiful Mornin'.' My most consistent song through the ride, though, has been a personal variation on 'To Dream the Impossible Dream,' substituting 'ride' for 'fight' and, of course 'Nan' for 'man,' always trying to reach the unreachable star!"

🐾 🐾 🐾 🐾 🐾

Many people congratulated me on finishing the ride and told me I should be proud. Instead of pride, I feel thankful this avenue has opened for me and potentially for thousands of other people to take charge of our lives and to live such an impossible dream. Jay thanked me for my spirit and advocacy. I thanked him for giving me the means to save my life. Not everyone with Parkinson's can ride across Iowa. But everyone can do their best to make their own version of this story. There is no hero award for sitting on a bike for hours on end. (Aching bottom? YES!)

Four of us with Parkinson's rode in our group: John, Jim, Mark, and I. These fabulous men are fabulous not because they rode 450 miles, but because they opened their experiences to the world with the hope of impacting others. And they surely pulled me along on the harder days.

I can't say enough about Jay, both for his research and his humble self. Most of all, I know I couldn't have done this without Doug. In nearly 40 years of marriage, we have never encountered anything like this PD challenge. He knows what I need—encouragement or a kick in the butt—and doesn't hesitate to provide either.

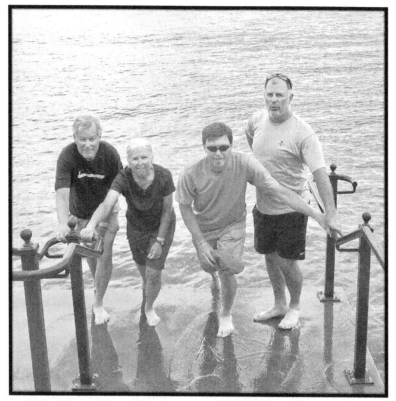

Tired toes in the Mississippi
Doug, Nan, John and Phil

Chapter 10. RAGBRAI Energy

After RAGBRAI, Doug and I fished our way home. In order to keep on cycling we put our bikes on the back of our little van and stowed a bike trainer inside, allowing me to spin for an hour nearly every day even if there was not a paved road or a bike path to ride on. Typically I would set up my trainer by a beautiful river, scope out fishing places as I pedaled, then don my waders and harass trout the rest of the day. Each time I pedaled, it felt like I was plugging my charger into the wall, giving me plenty of energy for wading and casting. We laughed, "First I bike; and then I fish!"

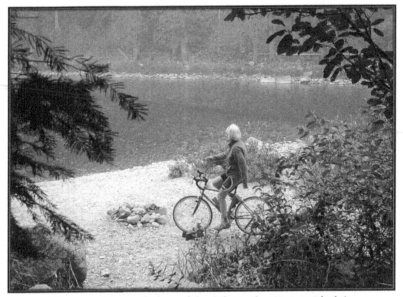

Streamside training ride (Photo by Doug Little)

Back home, at my fall doctor's visit, I received a great bill of health again, enabling me to reduce my dose of Requip XL from 8 to 6 mg per day. I continued with 1 mg of Azilect and added 0.5 mg of clonazepam to help with my newly diagnosed REM sleep behavior disorder. (I describe this diagnosis later, in the chapter "REM Sleep Behavior Disorder.") With the meds and cycling, I was pretty close to fully functional. My hand shook now and then, but not much.

Unexpectedly I developed a new role and purpose in life, acting as a resource as friends and doctors referred newly diagnosed PwPs to me as someone who had been there, and was still coming to grips with this disease. Sharing the story of Jay's research and the results I had experienced somehow enabled me to gain some control over my life.

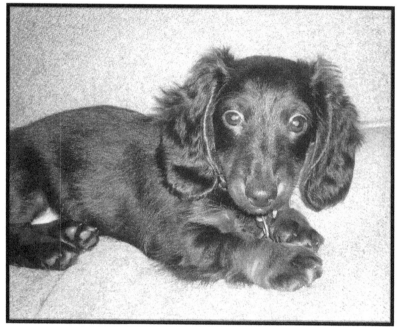

Lincoln as puppy (Photo by Doug Little)

Another diversion engaged our family. After the loss of Jester, it didn't take long for us to realize the holes in our hearts could indeed be filled by a new puppy. Although we both had agreed to wait, when I saw a picture online of a dog that looked hauntingly like Jester, I was compelled to call the breeder to see if perhaps she had a puppy for sale. Astonishingly enough, this woman had originally bred Jester and had sold him to her friend, who had sold him to us! Jester's mom still lived with her. When she heard our story, Jester's step-nephew, Lincoln, joined our family and his cousin, Addie, on the last day of 2009.

Chapter 11. Establishing PFP Classes

After RAGBRAI 2009 I continued to enjoy excellent health while riding nearly every day at the high cadence pace of 80–90 rpm, either outdoors or indoors on my trainer. Iowa had put a lot of energy in my storage tank. My hand tremor and all my other Parkinson's symptoms were seldom apparent. I realized cycling would be a part of the rest of my life. How fortunate to be able to do something I loved to make me and keep me well!

When others heard about my experience, I received a request in December 2009 from a local hospital asking me to help set up a tandem cycling class for Parkinson's patients based on Jay Alberts' protocols. I was delighted. People added resources from all quarters: R+E Cycles made four custom tandems at cost, paid for by generous donors who had connections to cycling or Parkinson's or both; Jay Alberts sent all the extras; the American Parkinson Disease Association became the conduit for donations; and a group of wonderful women quickly became the organizing force for the new program. Everyone gained inspiration and energy from the four selected participants who couldn't wait to begin. I hoped and prayed some of these People with Parkinson's would have experiences even partly similar to mine.

I had been given a huge gift, a means to be proactive about my disease, which I hoped would be shared by other PwPs.

Doug and I had to leave for RAGBRAI 2010 before the first eight-week-long tandem cycling class for PD patients began, but we kept in close touch with the coordinator while we were gone. My heart was at the opening class even though my body was in Iowa. Fabulous volunteers called "captains" powered the tandems on the front, while the four PwPs rode on the backs of the tandems as "stokers." Our PwPs ranged from those who were fairly healthy to a woman who had had four Deep Brain Stimulation (DBS) surgeries (electrodes were implanted in her brain to help her function more normally) and had never ridden a bike. Our goal was to have them riding at 80–90 rpm by the end of the second week. All of them were riding at or above the target goal on the first day. Our team leader reported how emotional and joyful the PwPs felt, celebrating that, with this cycling class, they might experience some relief from their PD symptoms.

The hospital eagerly awaited results, hoping to bolster their efforts to find resources to sustain the project. The most important issue from the hospital's perspective was whether or not Parkinson's symptoms actually would be alleviated through the cycling, thereby justifying their investment. The next issue was determining how forced-exercise cycling would affect the PwPs' cognition and emotional health. ("Forced exercise" refers to the cadence, or revolutions per minute, of 80–90 rpm. An average PwP normally cycles at 55–60 rpm.)

Initial reports indicated the class was making a profound difference in the lives of the PwPs. Although many questions remained, the PwPs had a great feeling of finally being able to do something proactive about a disease that, prior to this, could be addressed only through medications, and that could be put on hold only now and then through various forms of exercise.

Even after the first week, the organizers from the hospital and the volunteers made extensive notes on how to replicate the program in other venues. Getting the class off the ground was one thing. Sustaining the program, and seeing to what extent it worked with patients at all levels of the disease, would be huge questions to address. There was so much more to learn before we considered sharing a "how to" with the rest of the world.

However, as word of the success of Jay Alberts' program spread, people from all over the United States contacted him for help in setting up their own tandem programs. He often referred them to me, so what had begun as a hospital class became a pilot for what might be a national dissemination system for PFP programs.

At that point we had no licensing agreement, and therefore nothing more than goodwill binding people to the main protocols of the program as identified by Dr. Alberts: maintain 80 to 90 rpm (the cadence range), ensure that patients wear heart-rate monitors, and make sure they stay within 60 to 85 percent of their maximum heart rate. I returned from RAGBRAI 2010, eager to see the class in action and experience for myself the many successes I had heard about; unfortunately, the class I saw was not the class I expected. PwPs were not using heart rate monitors, and some captains had their patients spinning at up to 120 rpm. I asked questions and was told to leave. This was far from the homecoming I had expected.

We had nowhere to go but up. That would take a while.

Chapter 12. Fishing and Tremors

I told myself at the beginning of my sojourn with Parkinson's that I didn't intend to have the disease define my life even though it would inevitably necessitate adjustments along the way. I didn't want to live just to be alive. Hopefully I could still be active! Wending our way to Iowa, we first drove to West Yellowstone, fishing every day and enjoying the wonders of the park, reconnecting with old friends and making new ones along the way.

A highlight of our time in Yellowstone was spending a few days with the Yellowstone Volunteer Fly-Fishing Program, sponsored by Patagonia and run by the aptly named, ever-upbeat seasonal park ranger, Tim Bywater. We were to fish Trout Lake in the north of the park, trying to catch hybrid cutthroat and rainbow trout for a research study. Eager to begin, I dashed up the steep quarter-mile trail to the lake, oblivious to any Parkinson's symptoms. On this perfectly still day with not a ripple on the water, several fishermen cast from the shore and two men paddled around in float tubes but no one had had a strike by the time we arrived.

Hundreds of big fish crowded the shores; they just weren't biting. Although it was tempting to cast to those fish, Tim assured us it would be a waste of time. He told me to cast my fly as far as I could, then ignore it for at least ten minutes. He cast his fly, put his rod on the shore, and lay down in the grass! Patience is not one of my virtues, but I tried. Pretty soon I caught the first fish of the day, a 14-inch rainbow, not a huge catch but the only one so far. Then a guy in a float tube yelled that he saw bicolored ants on the water. I changed my fly, fingers working just fine, and cast again. Quickly a fish gulped it and we were on our way. Although it took a long time to land, I caught my largest fish ever, a bright, beautiful 24-inch rainbow. It was so fat I could not hold it for a picture after the weighing, measuring and fin-clipping had taken place. We laughed as it swam freely away.

Buoyed by success, I cast the bicolored ant again on the still water. Almost immediately another fish gobbled it up. Already exhausted from landing the first trout, when the second fish took off I could barely hold the rod. It was another big fish, but adrenaline trumps exhaustion. I tried to reel in the slack whenever I could, which was seldom. The fish ran out nearly

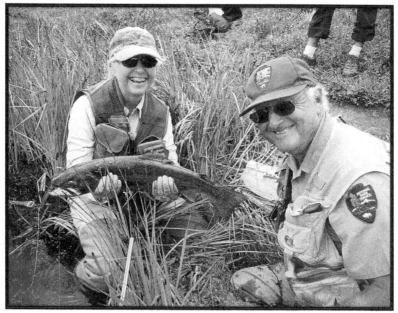

Trout Lake rainbow at Yellowstone
with Ranger Tim Bywater
(Photo by Doug Little)

all my line, even the backing. Then the line went slack and we all moaned. Another "one that got away" story. Oh well, it was a fun run. I reeled in slowly, arm aching, hand nearly paralyzed, until abruptly the line moved! Fish still on! Everyone started whooping and hollering as I awkwardly landed it. I had no idea which of us was more exhausted, the fish or me. Landing that 21-inch rainbow helped me realize I have a lot more capacity to draw on than I thought possible.

A premier fishing shop in West Yellowstone, Blue Ribbon Flies, published an article about the Yellowstone Volunteer Fly-Fishing Program along with a photo of Tim, me, and the 21-inch rainbow. Big smiles all around. Daughter Jodie said I'm famous—well, less than famous, but it was fun.

The next day we awoke to a layer of fresh snow on the mountains. As we started walking slowly across the Lamar Valley toward the river, bearing right to avoid a herd of buffalo munching along our usual path, we noticed a black grizzly further to our right. We stood quietly for about twenty minutes watching the drama unfold, hoping we wouldn't be an integral part of it. Tourists along the roadside had their binoculars on us as well as on the animals. Finally the buffalo caught scent of the bear and moved further away from us. The bear got interested in some pronghorn in the other direction and ambled off. We smiled, enjoyed the wildflowers, eagle and osprey above, a little chick lost from its mama in the tall grass and the antics of a mother mallard pretending to be injured to lure us away from her nest. Not many fish, but plenty of drama. Better than watching a National Geographic special, we were in it. The drama had focused so much of my attention I stopped shaking.

Still heading to Iowa, on our way to Soda Butte in the Lamar Valley we passed two grizzlies and two wolves competing for a buffalo carcass still partly in the river. Tens of ravens filled nearby trees, waiting their turn. Look for the ravens to find the kill. Yellowstone's Lamar Valley: the Serengeti of North America. Little did I know that in the not too distant future, courtesy of Parkinson's disease, I would be in the African Serengeti. Hundreds of tourists took photos of the grizzlies, wolves and disappearing buffalo. At Soda Butte we found few fish, but wildflowers bloomed everywhere. At one point we climbed over a rise and found ourselves at eye level with a field of blue lupine, yellow flowers, pink geraniums, sweet peas and clover. Sometimes I weep at beauty.

🐟 🐟 🐟 🐟 🐟

The long days of fishing brought a surprising change in my hand/arm tremors. Usually I had a hard time falling asleep because I constantly patted myself. Even though I tried to bury the offending hand under a pillow or body part, it took a long time for me to drift off. When I awoke, the patting started again, sometimes keeping me awake for the rest of the night. However, since I had been fly-fishing several hours a day, the night and morning tremors were greatly reduced, sometimes even gone. I wondered if the repetitive casting action mitigated the tremors. Cycling is also repetitive action. Perhaps there is a correlation. Maybe we should start Fly-Fishing for Parkinson's.

The really good news was that, through all those weeks in Yellowstone, I felt amazingly well. My finger dystonia stopped. I experienced no foot dystonia either and very little tremor in the night and morning. I'm not exactly sure why I was escaping the problems of Parkinson's, but I know anxiety is a huge issue in both the onset and the direction of the disease. When I could spend day after day essentially free of anxiety, with my most pressing worries being whether or not a fish would take my fly or if I would find a nice place to cycle, I was living a stress-free life. Possibly the lack of stress, coupled with the extensive outpouring of energy in exercise, made a huge difference in my Parkinson's. My personal take-away points: lower stress; increase exercise.

This improvement in symptoms was even more amazing since I had lowered my dose of Requip XL from 6 mg to 4 mg in February and was operating on the Requip, 1 mg of Azilect and 0.5 mg of clonazepam for my REM behavior disorder. Unexpectedly, I had been able to steadily reduce my medication while improving my health.

We were ready for RAGBRAI. There was nothing quite like going from relatively flat rides at sea level to pumping up and down steep hills at over 6,000 feet to get those muscles and lungs in shape. As always, when I couldn't ride on a road, I would amuse the masses by spinning on my trainer in a parking lot or alongside a highway or a river, each workout lasting for an hour at 80–90 rpm. I loved people's expressions when they saw a rider going nowhere on the side of the road. It was amazing there weren't any accidents.

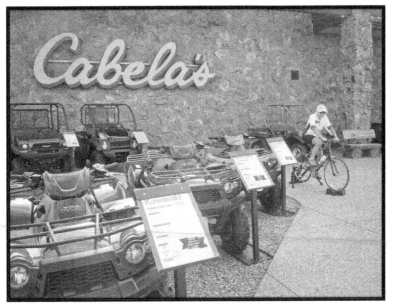

Training in Sidney, Nebraska
No trout stream available
(Photo by Doug Little)

Chapter 13. RAGBRAI 2010, July 25-31

I'm told there were 10,000 official RAGBRAI riders in 2010 with up to 15,000 riding on any one day. Of our PFP team of fifty riders, four of us had PD. The returning PD patient from last year, John, looked better and stronger than before. His posture was much different—more upright—and he looked ready to take on the world. We were a team. The new PD riders added quite a different dimension. One thirty-nine-year-old had been diagnosed for eight years. Three years ago he was

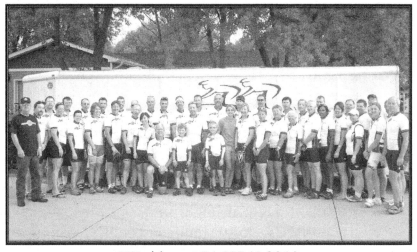

PFP riders at RAGBRAI 2010
(Photo by Doug Little)

using a cane full time. Then he started cycling and within weeks he was able to put away his cane and appear like a normal person most of the time. His experience was remarkable! If the three of us were in a group with non-PD patients, anyone would be challenged to pick us out. The other woman had suffered from PD for nineteen years and had had

DBS surgery on one side. She and her husband rode a tandem. It was hard, but this courageous couple pedaled their way across Iowa with the rest of us. One PwP rode a tandem, one rode a recumbent tandem, one rode a recumbent tricycle and I rode my bike.

Day 1: On the Road Again

"The first day of RAGBRAI 2010 brought back so many memories of last year, only this time without the fear factor. The first day's ride was supposed to be 69 miles, but it was considerably longer ... the story each day. It's hot here, seemed like 200 degrees the night before we started. But it was only about 100 (maybe 90). With adrenaline running high, the ride was a breeze. At one point, someone dropped a water bottle in the road, and the guy ahead of me unclipped his shoe and deftly kicked the bottle into the ditch. Many cheers. Later I learned a sixteen-year-old in our group was able to lean over and pick up a bottle at high speed! I was lucky just to stay on the bike. Iowa still has a lot of corn and beans!"

Day 2: The Importance of Knowing Who You Are

"We thought it might rain, but Monday dawned sunny, promising to be another scorcher. This was an 85-mile day, with fewer hills than on Sunday. With legs still pretty strong, it wasn't difficult.

"Success with RAGBRAI and Parkinson's is partly determined by eating properly. Having PD makes it particularly important that I pay attention to nutrition. We have cereal, V8 juice and coffee before setting out, then drink bottle after bottle of water supplemented with Vitalite but still don't have much to show for it when we go to the bathroom. At about 20-30 miles we start to eat, trying to throw in some protein along with the inevitable pie and the last treat of the day, Beekman's Homemade Ice Cream. Just like last year, nearly everyone from PFP stops at Beekman's.

"Connections are being made. As we ride along wearing our Pedaling For Parkinson's jerseys, people invariably ask what the program is about; they comment about Jay's talks on the radio or TV; they tell us about a friend or relative with the disease or just talk. Hours go by for each of us as we share the PFP story, inspiring others to try the same.

"Monday evening a farmer and his wife drove 60 miles to talk about the program with Jay and those of us with street credibility. The young, perfectly healthy farmer had fallen off a ladder and gone into a coma and when he awoke, he had Parkinson's. He was so depressed he wasn't sure why he kept on living. His wife was absolutely distraught. As we spoke, I asked about his history: What had he done so far in life? Who was he? He told me he had been captain of all the teams in high school, a leader in his community, a successful farmer. People had looked up to him; they had always looked up to him; now they looked at him not knowing what to say. He felt he had nothing to offer either his community or his wife.

"Knowing that stories make truths tangible, I told him about Joe, a psychiatrist friend of ours, who lives in Philadelphia. We visited Joe shortly after my diagnosis, after a hiatus of over thirty years. Almost immediately he asked what was wrong—not physically, but in my heart. What was I afraid of? I told him I feared I had lost my identity when I started taking pills for Parkinson's. Was the real me still there or was I just a construct of drugs?

"Joe told us of an experience that had happened to him at a conference of psychiatrists. When participants were asked to introduce themselves, they went around the room describing their specialties in psychiatry, but when his turn came, he simply said, 'I am Joe.' Confused, people asked what he meant. They wanted to know what he did, not who he was, but they had asked who he was and he didn't consider his identity to be what he did at work. If you wanted to know Joe, you had to take the time to learn who he was.

"He assured me the essential Nan was still there. I had not and would not lose my identity because I have Parkinson's and I take medications. The characteristics I have, good and bad, may be exacerbated by this condition, but a whole new me will not emerge. As I felt a huge weight drop off my back, I realized I had been as afraid of the medications as of the disease. Like the farmer, I had been afraid my core self was gone and I was worried that what was left was not worth much.

"As I told my story about Joe to the farmer and his wife, I watched the weight drop from him as well. He realized his essential character was still there and he had much to give to his community as well as to his family. Opening this door for others reminds me to keep it open for myself."

Day 3: Roads and Heat

"Day three always seems challenging. It's no longer the first exciting day. It's no longer the second day when your legs still have energy. It's the *third day*, when your body screams, 'What is this about!' What is it about? I have observed that much of life is about meeting challenges and making stories, and this is no different.

"Today's ride was a mere 66 miles, a piece of cake. We started a little later, 7:20 a.m. instead of the early 6:40 a.m. start the day before, thinking we would zoom through it. Out of cereal, we shared the group donuts, not a great idea for sure. Pie for breakfast? I think I ate pie and donuts! Then two bananas, tons of water with rehydration powder, probably six or seven bottles. More pie! What was I thinking? Obviously nothing related to health. I paid the price as my constipated body tried to rid itself of the unaccustomed 'foods'.

"I waited in the air-conditioned library to go to the bathroom, along with a half-hour line of others who couldn't face a hot Honey Bucket. It didn't matter if we had to go. The air conditioner grabbed us and held us there.

"As I stood there in the library basement in distress, my phone rang, 'Ode to Joy', on the loudest setting. Everyone laughed while I fumbled through my jersey pockets. Prior to leaving for Iowa my quilting friend, Carol, from West Yellowstone had talked me into buying raffle tickets for a beautiful poppy wall hanging she had made for a fundraiser for the West Yellowstone Historical Center. I won the wall hanging! I squealed and shared the good news with all my curious new friends waiting in line. Who would guess? The next day as I was riding along (properly fed), a woman pulled up next to me shouting, 'I know you! You're the woman who won the quilt in the bathroom!'

"Wind had promised to be our friend, wafting cool breezes, but instead hot blasts came at us crosswise. Road surfaces were often laced with tar filled cracks, or partly filled with tar. At one point, when a young man directly in front of me caught his tire in a crack, the abrupt stop threw him splat on the highway. If I had been ten feet closer, I would have run right over him. As it was, I was wary and had maintained enough open space to avoid tragedy for both of us.

"Rural roads in Iowa have rumbles, strips of corrugated concrete that warn drivers a stop sign is just ahead. Three bike-jarring stretches of rumbles precede each stop sign. Cyclists scream, 'Rumbles!' to warn other riders. It's a wonder there aren't more rumble accidents. Near the end of today's ride, when everyone was sunburned beyond recognition and riders audibly wondered, 'Why are we doing this?', the road turned, sending us directly into the wind for several miles. Slow, slow, slow. But we knew that during the next stretch the wind would be crosswise, at least not in our faces. We turned off the well-paved, headwind road onto a raggedy rumble that lasted for miles. Hands and butts took a beating until finally the town appeared, and the ride was only 7 miles longer than advertised.

"After a few false turns (what a surprise!) I finally found 'our' house and rolled into the front yard to cheers and greetings. Never mind I was one of the last to arrive; it was great! Doug and I got our swimsuits and walked over to the nearby retirement home for a glorious play in the pool. Some men had come to hear from PD patients about the program, so I sat with the others and discussed it all with them before heading out to dinner, capping another fine day after all!"

Day 4: A New Day, Temperatures Dropped

"We learned yesterday's high was 113 degrees in the sun, with a median air temperature of over 98. No wonder we all died on the vine. But last night an intense storm blew through, quickly dumping buckets of water, waking everyone. Some folks spent an hour or two securing their tents and contemplated seeking shelter. Everyone held ground, however, and no one suffered anything more than loss of sleep. Doug and I woke up briefly, noted the storm and promptly returned to oblivion. Apparently the lightning and thunder were nearly simultaneous, but we knew nothing. The net result of all of this excitement was the temperature dropped about 20 degrees. It was still in the 80s, but after the day before, not a problem.

"We met in the morning at 7:00 for our group photo, and then we rode off to conquer the 55 miles. Heavy clouds blocked the sun as a light breeze encouraged us in our pedaling. Having stocked up on cereal and milk, we had a normal healthy breakfast, powering us with the right kind of energy. With such a short ride, I didn't even stop for the first 20 miles except to walk my bike through each crowded town along with the swarms of riders. Walking is good, both for sharing the entertainment and culture of the various towns and for resting specific body parts.

"This leg of the ride was notable for a paucity of Honey Buckets. Mile after mile with no Honey Buckets meant my life became increasingly difficult. No respite in sight, I finally asked a woman at a stand if she had a place I could use. She pointed to the cornfield. Oh my. The cornfield was surrounded by barbed wire, more of a challenge than I was willing to attempt. But there was a handy *silo!* City girl meets silo. Whew! I finally felt like I had crossed a barrier and was truly part of the RAGBRAI group. Perhaps most important was the realization I could squat for an extended time (constipation again) without getting leg cramps. Parkinson's patients face endless uncharted challenges.

"Our Pedaling For Parkinson's jerseys continued to provoke interest and encouragement. I rode about 15 miles with one man who has the disease, and by the end of our talk I believe he had hope. I thought he was doing pretty well already, but could see he felt depressed and alone. No longer. When I got to camp (at the local hospital), Doug already had people waiting to talk with me. After they left, another woman appeared. Then a man I met the day before. On and on it goes. One big answer to Why *are* we doing this, anyway? is that so many people want/need to know this concept works and they can in fact take charge of their own lives. What a gift to be able to give!

"Tomorrow is 85 miles. I'm feeling good and hoping the big gears on my bike will pull me down the road."

Day 5: Riding Through Pain

"The day started out great: good weather, good temperature and no pain while riding, just in my butt when I was off the bike. Seventy-two miles to go. Brimming with overconfidence, I gave in yet again to the sugar syndrome. Glazed donut at 6:30 a.m., first pie by 8:00 a.m., more pie, ear of corn dripping with butter, ice cream and not enough water. No protein at all. As the first 30 miles went fine, my silliness increased, followed by the inevitable meltdown. Sad story. I ran into Rene from our PFP group who was in a similar state. We rode together for many miles, giving me the chance to learn about her life and her faith and to be supported by her remarkable self. We stopped at PB&J when we thought we had 20 miles to go, where fortunately we ran into Doug who had figured out a direct route: just 6 more miles to ride. Happily Rene could read a map, so we pulled each other in to home base.

"Jay gave his talk to the Iowa chapter of the American Parkinson Disease Association, preceded by a great chicken dinner provided by the group. I enjoyed hearing his story yet again and being brought up to date on the most recent news on the program.

"Unfortunately it was difficult for me to concentrate. From the beginning of the ride I've had a persistent pain in my butt. Neither standing nor sitting eased the stabbing sensations, causing me to nearly cry more than once. Our masseuse did her best, to little avail. Later in the evening Doug used a rolling pin-like gadget to work on the site, which improved things tremendously. I expect it was a herniated disc.

"This was raffle night as well. As before, every fifty dollars we raised for PFP earned us one raffle ticket. Jay spread out the treasures to be raffled off, and we all allocated our tickets as we wished in each container next to a desired item. After the drawings Doug and I came back with more jerseys, a bike computer, new pants for me, and a pink bike bell! Can hardly wait to use the bell.

"Other than the leg, which only hurt when I was on my feet or sitting, which meant all the time, it was a very good day."

Day 6: Complain About Heat: You Get Rain!

"Today began with a heavy overcast and much discussion about whether we should take jackets. Fortunately, Doug and I did. Although they shed not a drop of the downpour, they did help keep us a bit warm when the heavens opened almost immediately after we hit the road. This was not gentle Seattle rain. For four and a half hours we rode through a downpour so heavy I found it difficult to see through my glasses. Since my rearview mirror was attached to my glasses, if I took the glasses off, I had no rearview mirror, plus the rain hit my eyeballs now and then. Painful drops also hit the sunburn blisters along my lower lip. Rain in Iowa comes with thunder and lightning, lots of it. Each time the lightning flashed, I counted. The closest boomed just four counts after the lightning, sounding like the gods intended to do us all in. I kept on pedaling. I liked the cool; I passed the pie stands and continued to drink lots of water laced with Vitalyte."

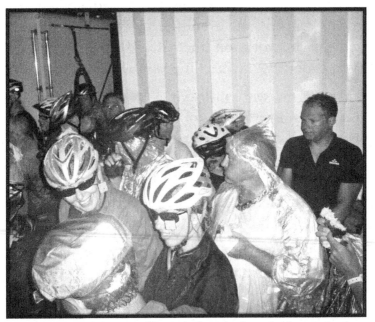

RAGBRAI riders seeking shelter in handy farm shed after stopping at Mr. Pork Chop (Photo by Doug Little)

"At the beginning of the day nearly all the children were riding, most on tandems with parents. When the lightning flashed too close, parents decided to 'sag' all the kids, opting to put the kids and their bikes into whatever vehicles were available. Many of our adults wanted out too, some because of the intense weather, others because they didn't have jackets and were approaching hypothermia. Adults sagged in the

PFP truck, and Susie drove our van filled with the children, bringing everyone safely to the campsite. Definitely a dramatic day!

"Doug came through for me yet again. Part of the ride was into the wind and the rain, and I was running low on steam. He rode in front of me so I could draft the last hour, first through the rain and then when the sun came out for the last half hour. He has a great way of glancing at me and knowing what I need to make it through. Perhaps I might have gotten to the end without drafting, but I surely would have been more of a basket case.

"One PD compatriot was already asleep when we arrived after having suffered a bike breakdown this day and extreme fatigue the day before. She didn't ride the whole way, but her ride was a success beyond measure. What an inspiration! A woman with nineteen years of PD and DBS surgery on one side of her brain, she not only tried RAGBRAI but, with the help of her patient, determined husband, completed nearly all of it.

"Several of us went out to dinner to discuss how to translate Jay's research into classes for PD patients. Nothing is set in concrete, but good questions are on the table.

"One thing on my mind is a disconnect of sorts between those of us in the group who have PD and the others, some of whom know a great deal about PD and some who are either too shy to ask or who have never been told. I suggested to Jay it would be helpful to initiate a discussion in which anyone could ask us anything. The group agreed, so we had a large circle with three of us ready to answer questions. Very much like a Native American talking circle, this format gave permission for anyone to ask questions and for others to listen in, hearing answers to things they might be hesitant to ask. We went well into dark, and many people thanked us afterward for opening our experiences to them. For those of us with PD, it was a high point of the week.

"During the circle one of the children whispered to me that his dad didn't feel well. I told him to tell Doug and soon I noticed Doug, Jay and Barry, our MD, quietly easing out of the circle. I learned later our fabulous trailer driver, Jason Moser, overall *make it happen* guy, was taken to the hospital with kidney stones. His son Keaton had stepped forward, confident this group would take care of both his dad and him. He was right.

"Oddly enough, rain and all, again it was a very good day."

Day 7: Potter's Hill

"Still suffering with my hip/butt pain, I felt exhausted at the start of the day. Although the ride was only 51 miles, my sense of unease was exacerbated by concern about the frequently referenced Potter's Hill that lay ahead. All week long we had heard demonizing stories about Potter's Hill, the infamous *last big hill* on the 2010 RAGBRAI. In pioneer days, Potter's Field was a place to die—a place to be buried unknown, unsung, unmarked. How many people climbing Potter's Hill today would feel like they were headed for Potter's Field?

"Potter's Hill, the entrance to Dubuque, is 1 mile long with an average grade of 6 percent. Think of the interstate highways that advise trucks to use the right lane while going up a 6 percent grade and provide a runaway-truck ramp for those who lose their brakes on a 6 percent downgrade. One mile at 6 percent. Reportedly tucked in the 1 mile is 0.25 mile at 15-19 percent. The roof grade on an Iowa farmhouse is 25 percent. When I bought my cycle in Seattle in the mid-1990s, they assured me the gearing was so good I could climb a telephone pole. I was about to discover just how good that gearing was.

"Strategy. I knew if I rode quickly down the inevitable hill before Potter's, I could get a head start on the big one, which might help a little. As I crested the hill before Potter's, I realized a new strategy was clearly in order. Below me, at the base of the hill, thousands of riders were clumped up, packing the road handlebar to handlebar, wheel to wheel. Many riders were already walkers or fallers, having given up before even starting the climb. At first I thought I would see parts of the roadway through a dense tree cover, but actually I could see no roadway at all, just bursts of colorful jerseys still packed tightly together. So, instead of flying down the hill, I descended gripping my brakes, willing myself to be one of the few riders who would ride all the way to the top. Parkinson's never entered my mind. No room for trivia.

"My memory of the ride up Potter's Hill is blurred. Getting through the mob of walkers provided a major challenge. A woman in purple, *purple* Lycra walked her bike in front of me in the middle of the road. Most of us wear black to draw the eyes away from the seat to the jersey, but she had the seat and the guts to wear purple. I yelled, '*Purple Pants, move to your right!*' The crowd took up the chant. *Purple Pants, move to your right!* She moved; I kept pedaling. I heard a yell behind me. *Emergency dismount! So sorry!* The hapless rider crashed directly behind me, followed by who-knows-how-many falling around him like dominoes.

"At first I could ride steadily, if slowly. I heard someone on my left calling out degrees of incline . . . 4 . . . 6 . . . 8 . . . 11. I didn't hear anything after 11. He probably had no extra energy for the numbers game. An 11 percent grade is Tour de France stuff, and most of us were decidedly not Tour de Anything material.

"I keep a list of friends and donors in the little tool bag under my bicycle seat. Whenever I'm having a tough time, for whatever reason, I mentally scroll through the list and feel my supporters willing me through the challenge. I thought of these supporters and silently repeated their names. One of my friends is Evelyne. She and her husband have ridden from Seattle to Patagonia, nearly around the world, and from Hanoi to Ho Chi Minh City. They know how to ride. To maximize each pedal stroke, she taught me to keep continuous pressure on both feet at all times, pushing down and pulling up. Into my mind popped 'Evelyne . . . Up . . . Evelyne . . . Up,' over and over the same phrase. She was the only one who made it out of my bike bag into my conscious brain that day. I actually passed people with my pulling/pushing stroke. I was afraid if I quit I would just fall over, knock over those behind me and probably get hurt.

"I dared to glimpse at my heart-rate monitor and looked away . . . 147. My maximum heart rate is supposed to be 155. I always assumed (with no real knowledge, of course) that over 155 meant heart attack. The number climbed as my energy waned.

"Someone on the sidelines screamed we were almost there. I could see plenty of uphill to go and knew there was at least one liar in Iowa. As we were at the end of the 19 percent grade and my heart-rate monitor registered 166, I wasn't dead or close to dead. My legs didn't scream, but I could feel a massive thumping in my chest. When the incline flattened a bit, numbers on my heart-rate monitor slowly dropped. The only time I heard anyone swear in all seven days of RAGBRAI was at the top of Potter's Hill. 'Well, that was a bitch,' someone muttered quietly. No one argued. Potter's Hill is not something I'll try again.

"To add insult to injury, Potter's Hill was followed by about ten Sons and Daughters of Potter's. Most people got off at the top of Potter's, but, mistakenly believing we must be almost to the Mississippi, I kept on pedaling, asking other riders if we weren't really close. No one knew.

"We were not close. After an eternity, eventually I could see the Mississippi and soon I could pick out our van in the parking lot surrounded by swarms of people and cycles. Our group cheered as I rode in. Particularly after the circle the night before, I felt so close to everyone. Riders leaped forward, taking many photos. When the group heard I had ridden all the way up Potter's, they were incredulous. I felt a bit incredulous myself. The power of community and support is beyond description.

"I was told I was the only PD person in our group to ride the entire distance. Didn't matter. More than anything, I'm grateful I could do it. The ride would not have been possible without Doug, ably assisted by many others along the way. (He was dubbed Nan's Domestique, which in cycling parlance means a bicycle racer who works for the benefit of his team and team leader.)

"We dipped our bike wheels in the Mississippi and returned to find a TV reporter waiting to interview People with Parkinson's. My friend and teammate, John,

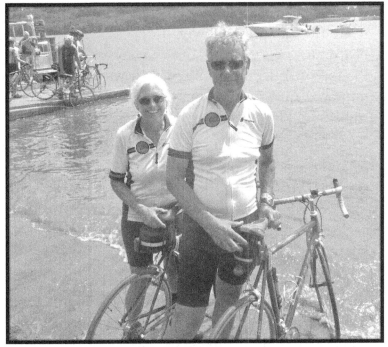

Wheels in the Mississippi
RAGBRAI 2010

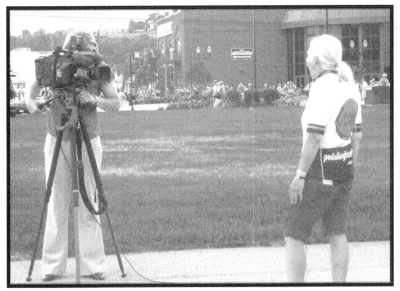

"Airtime" Nan in Dubuque
(Photo by Doug Little)

spoke with her for a long time, sincerely pouring out his heart, lacing his comments with clever witticisms she didn't understand. While I was being interviewed, I noticed the cameraman panning down to photograph my shaking hand. I was on the evening news, shaking hand and all, but there was no mention of John. I told him he has to learn how to shake if he wants to be on the news. After Doug gave me the moniker 'Airtime' and called John 'Floortime', John added to the laughter by mockingly referring to the reporter as Diane Sawyer's Second Cousin's Niece."

🂓 🂓 🂓 🂓 🂓

I felt great about RAGBRAI 2010. Through miles and miles of riding I thought of little more important than cracks in the road, other riders' behavior, corn and beans, lush landscapes, friendly Iowans and friendly riders. I never heard anger or road rage. How could thousands of riders spend an exhausting week together on two-lane roads without strife? The tone was set to encourage each other, not compete. Everyone who rode at all accomplished something, and we all supported each other in our quests. Lightning, thunder, heat, accidents, all brought us closer together. It's can be a dangerous undertaking. When two men collided, one died. We all understand and respect the ride.

I enjoyed people asking questions about PD and registering amazement that I ride to improve my health. I loved the time with Jay and his amazing family, and with the other families. I marveled at the nine-year-old who rode the entire RAGBRAI on his own bike, whizzing past me every day. Most of all I loved being with Doug, knowing he watches me from the corner of his eye and will respond if I need help, even when I don't know I need it.

Once our friends were gone and the crowds dispersed, we drove to the Field of Dreams where Doug got to play ball. His turn. Finally. I slept ten hours.

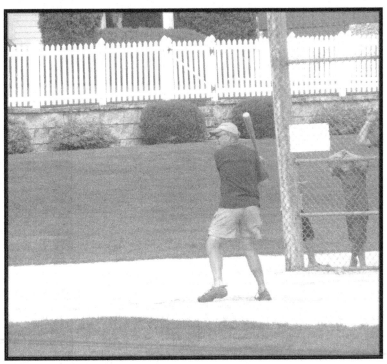

Doug at the Field of Dreams

Chapter 14. Mount Kilimanjaro: Background

In mid-September 2010, after our second RAGBRAI, I heard from noted Movement Disorder Specialist Dr. Monique Giroux's physician's assistant, Sierra Farris, asking if I knew anyone with PD who might want to climb 19,340-foot Mount Kilimanjaro the following July, joining a group of people with multiple sclerosis and Parkinson's disease. Sierra had heard

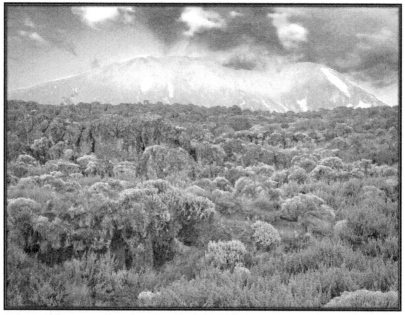

Kilimanjaro from the trail in (Photo by Doug Little)

a talk given by Lori Schneider of Empowerment Through Adventure who, burdened with MS, had climbed the Seven Summits (the highest peak on each continent, including Mount Everest). When Sierra heard that Lori was putting together a climb of Mount Kilimanjaro for people with MS to show the world that people with neurodegenerative diseases need not be constrained from living their dreams, she asked if some PwPs could go along as well. Having heard about my rides across Iowa, Sierra thought I might either be interested in Kilimanjaro myself or have suggestions of other PwPs who might want to go.

Eventually the group would be comprised of four pairs of people representing Parkinson's and ten representing MS. Most pairs included one person with an illness and another supporting the neurologically-challenged person.   All of us derived inspiration from Lori, our leader on this Leap of Faith climb.   She had shown through her personal example that people with neurodegenerative diseases are capable of far more than they expect.

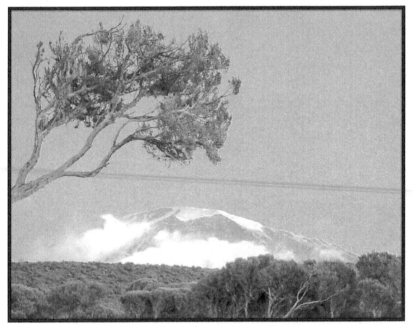

Kilimanjaro from the trail out
(Photo by Doug Little)

Sierra needed to find one or two fit PwPs who would be willing and able to join the adventure; both she and Dr. Giroux, would be going. Tempted, I told her I would try to think of other capable PwPs. I wrote to John Carlin, our buddy from RAGBRAI, and before we knew it, plans were setting in concrete. Doug and I, and John and his wife, Martha, would join the group. Subsequently two more spots opened up that Sierra filled with her own PD patients.

I felt honored to be invited to participate in this Leap of Faith. Having never climbed a mountain before, it certainly would be a leap for me.

Chapter 15. Mount Kilimanjaro: Training and Life

Concerned about the best way to train for the Kilimanjaro climb, we turned to our cycling friend Dorothy Baetz, who is a close friend of Mary Lou Wickwire, wife of noted mountain climber Jim Wickwire. Jim had one word for us: steps. He said steps, so steps it was. Seattle is noted for hills and lots and lots of steps. We live near the Howe Street stair climb on the west side of Capitol Hill. Climbing down the 388 steps, the view across Lake Union to the Space Needle and Queen Anne hill beyond is breathtaking. With boats, seaplanes and ever-changing patterns in the sky, it was always worth the effort.

At the apparent bottom, across the street and under the freeway . . . more steps. At the bottom of the 388, there was nowhere to go but back up, this time looking at the hillside plantings and gardens. Each day looked slightly different, sort of like the Indian stories that changed a little each time you heard them. When we got to the top, we turned around and did it again, and then again, and then again.

We used our first hill climbs to break in our new boots. Although I didn't carry a pack, I found it helpful to use my hiking staffs. Then I added my new pack with very little weight, adding more each time we climbed: 2 pounds, 4 pounds, 8 pounds, 10 pounds, up to 25 pounds. Doug kept adding too, up to 35 pounds. We discussed how many times to go up and down. It seemed like a good idea to just try it once or twice. Then, as we realized we were going to be climbing for hours and hours on end, carrying at least 15 to 25 pounds, we puffed and panted until we could go up and down those 388 steps five times with weighted packs.

Lots of people train on the stairs. Many are headed up Mount Rainier, others participate in sports, and others just do it to stay in very good shape. Almost every time we went, we compared notes with people we had seen before. Several University of Washington Husky football players leaped up and down the steps, taking two at a time. One former professional dancer performed arabesques every few stairs. People—from the very young to those older than us—climbed sideways, backwards, and everyway but on their hands. One older woman who wore a weighted vest had been coming for years. Even though we live close to the Howe Street stairs, we took advantage of a book describing Seattle stair climbs to explore many opportunities. Finding more information online, we experimented with varying the view. But the steps were all pretty much the same. We hiked stairs for six months until the following July. I often alternated steps with cycling. When Wickwire said steps, we took him seriously.

♆ ♆ ♆ ♆ ♆

Of course, our goal was to climb a mountain, not hike up and down steps. With that in mind, we added mountain hiking, or at least steep hill climbing, to our agenda. One thing we couldn't add was altitude. Seattle, of course, is at sea level, and there was no way we could get to a point where we were starting at 6,000 or 8,000 feet. But we do have mountains; the Cascade Range is less than an hour away, and Mount Rainier frames the cityscape.

We contacted Monique and Sierra and arranged to climb Mount Si, a training mountain quite close by. They were in better shape than we, as well as twenty years younger, so Mount Si proved easier for them. No matter, it was an opportunity to get to know them and to put a few miles on our legs. It's not unusual for people in the Seattle area to do trail running on Mount Si, even on their lunch hours. I considered it challenging to hike—no running. I had a long way to go. Although we had hoped to do lots of training with Monique and Sierra, unfortunately with our busy lives we only took two training hikes together.

Sierra told us that she and Monique shared an uncommon disability: they both always got acute mountain sickness at 10,000 feet, as though they crossed a magic line and the headache appeared. I was amazed they wanted to climb Mount Kilimanjaro, 19,340 feet, when they knew they would have splitting headaches most of the time on the trail. I could not have done that. Never having been over 10,000 feet, I wondered what was in store for me.

There were plenty of opportunities for local hikes. Mount Si. Tiger Mountain. Mailbox Peak. Mount Rainier. Tiger Mountain was the local "anybody can do it" mountain. Even more than Mount Si, Tiger Mountain was the lunchtime workout for lots of people on the east side of Lake Washington, including many from the nearby Microsoft campus. My Seattle women's hiking group climbed it fairly often, but it was always a challenge for many of us. It was not quite as difficult as Mount Si, however, so Doug and I fit several Tiger Mountain trips into our training program.

Mailbox Peak posed a more difficult challenge. As one might expect, at the top there's a mailbox. People were supposed to sign in and write comments about their climb, but when we got there the box overflowed with junk. Actually getting to the mailbox proved a bit treacherous as we clambered over slippery snow-covered boulders, like climbing up giant, uneven icy steps. Since I'm just two inches over five feet, those giant steps stressed my body parts, particularly my thighs. Every time I went up and over a rock I mentally thanked Doug for pushing me to endure all those Howe Street steps. I considered Mailbox Peak extremely difficult, probably as challenging as any hike we would attempt. I felt sure it was probably as hard as climbing Mount Kilimanjaro. Naiveté is a wonderful thing. But ascending Mailbox helped prepare us for physical challenges that would come later.

Oddly enough, once again, the more I exercised, the less I noticed any Parkinson's symptoms. My balance was just fine, I experienced no rigidity, I moved relatively quickly and my tremor was barely noticeable. Focusing on something outside of myself that had short and long-term goals nearly erased my anxiety about the disease and hence erased many symptoms.

We contacted another member of our Kilimanjaro troop, Nathan Henwood, one of the two PwPs Sierra recruited after John and me, who blithely suggested a training climb to Camp Muir on Mount Rainier, at about 10,000 feet. I had climbed to Camp Muir nearly thirty years ago in the summertime—no snow—a distant memory. Muir on June 5, 2011 seemed like a good idea except for deep snow covering the trail. Snow, deep mushy snow, increased the degree of difficulty by about four. How was I to know? I was willing to try.

Nathan's Parkinson's symptoms were much more severe than mine. A young onset patient, he had already had DBS surgery to implant electrodes on both sides of his head. Despite the surgery, he still had difficulties with the jerky movements of dyskinesia and other cardinal Parkinson's symptoms. A tremendously strong man with the will of an ox, he cheered everyone along with his consistently positive attitude; he didn't seem to see obstacles in the way and chuckled his way through the most daunting situations. He loved photography as much as he loved mountain climbing and excelled at both. On our climb to Camp Muir, Nathan carried nearly fifteen pounds of camera equipment along with his pack. Struggling with my fifteen pounds, I thought he might be carrying fifty or more pounds on our Mount Kilimanjaro trek. If anyone could do it, I expected Nathan could.

As we started out, I recall thinking that this hike up Rainier in the snow wasn't so bad. If Doug went a little faster, Nathan went a little slower, but generally we stayed together.

Whenever I was flagging, one or the other encouraged me. I know either one of them could have raced up that mountain in half the time I took, but our goal was to ensure the team got to the top, and I was part of the team. I felt sure we would need that teamwork to conquer Mount Kilimanjaro. After hours of arduous hiking, stretching my legs to match my stride to the holes in the snow ahead of me, I could finally see Camp Muir. It looked very close. Looks deceive. Surely it was only a half hour away. But after an hour it was still a half hour away, and then yet another half hour. By the time we were actually close, I could hardly trust my eyes. But in getting there, we confirmed we have grit. It would take a lot of grit to get up Mount Kilimanjaro.

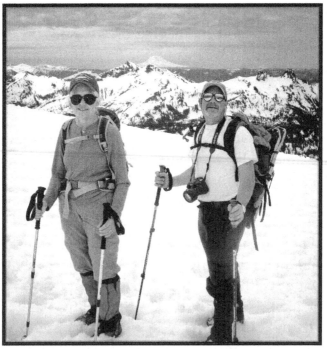

Training on Mount Rainier with Nathan
(Photo courtesy of Doug Little)

Our hike to Camp Muir occurred on a beautiful clear day. Nathan was really into his photography, so every now and then he would stop, turn around, and take a few photos. Although I looked and felt wasted, I pretended I was posing for a magazine photo shoot. We rested at Muir, sitting in snow, basking in the sun, getting a bit burned, and not caring a bit. Of course our legs were tired on the descent, and the snow was even mushier than in the morning. Every once in a while we found a stretch steep enough for sitting on our butts and glissading down, yelling like little kids. At the end of the day we were exhausted but happy with our new friendships. If nothing else happened on Kilimanjaro, at least Muir had brought Nathan into our lives.

Of course I had to keep up my cycling as well. Kilimanjaro would require a tremendous amount of energy, especially for me, energy that came from cycling. If I were to keep the PD beast at bay, I knew in my gut I had to continue pedaling as often as possible. To charge my internal batteries, Doug and I rode here and there around Lake Washington, each ride anywhere from eighteen to fifty miles. We rode trails and roads, sometimes together and sometimes separately. I convinced myself that unless my personal battery was fully charged through cycling I would never make it up Kilimanjaro, making my challenge as much mental as physical.

Varying the training regimen, we traveled several times to Vancouver, British Columbia. In Vancouver fabulous bike trails wind around all the waterways, through Stanley Park, past great shops and eateries and beyond. On one trip, Doug suggested an adventure: cycle from our downtown hotel out to Horseshoe Bay, eat lunch at our favorite fish-and-chips restaurant and return, a trip of over fifty miles—miles, not kilometers. Due to the winter Olympics in 2010, there had been massive road reconstruction, not all accurately reflected on maps. Our route took us around rocky headlands, along narrow two-lane roads past tastefully lavish mansions as well as more humble dwellings. It was a great day, except when we got a little lost and climbed a grueling incline, only to arrive at a cement barrier and a sign announcing the obvious: Road End. Only a little discouraged, we enjoyed the fast ride back down the incline and followed our noses back to the hotel. By that time, with very strong legs, even though sometimes the cycling was challenging, it was never impossible.

Like Seattle, Vancouver is built in the midst of lots of hills, home to three ski resorts and a demanding climb: the Grouse Grind. Tough. 29% average grade. Many steps. When

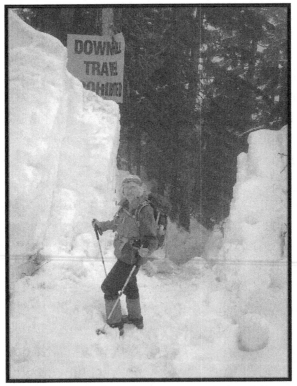

Grouse Grind, early season training hike
(Photo by Doug Little)

we arrived at the Grouse Grind, the trail was still buried in several feet of snow, a much greater challenge than we expected, but we had gaiters and hiking boots and hiking staffs, so we were ready to give it a shot. With the official entrance still closed for the season, we bushwhacked our way to a probable starting point. Alone, we scrambled to find a safe way up the generally hidden trail.

Grouse Grind reminded me of Mailbox Peak and its giant boulders, only with slippery logs as well. Neither of us is a mountain climber in the real sense of the word, knowing how to use pitons, axes and all the gear, but we do know that in order to move safely a climber must have a three-point touch, either two hands and a foot or two feet and a hand. I kept reminding myself about that as we slipped our way up the Grouse Grind, sometimes on the trail and sometimes cross-country, using shrubs as anchor points.

There's an aerial tramway at Grouse, so every once in a while we saw a carload of people gliding up the mountain on the enviable cable, toasty warm in their gondola. Near the top we met a work crew shoveling snow down the hill to open the trail. Imagine their surprise when we clambered over the final rocks and made it to the station without injury, two geri-active Yanks out for a day scramble in Vancouver. It was great! When I met Michael J. Fox many months later, our starting point of conversation was the Grouse Grind (followed immediately by a discussion of the Vancouver Canucks).

♃ ♃ ♃ ♃ ♃

When we rode across Iowa in RAGBRAI 2009 and 2010, I carried a list of my supporters. I liked keeping company with encouraging friends who shared a belief in my capacity to meet a challenge head-on and give it my all. Like plugging a lamp into a wall socket, the list gave me sustained energy.

Expanding the idea of encouragement further with Mount Kilimanjaro, I decided to ask friends and family to sign and send little scraps of material, maybe two inches by three inches, for me to sew together as my Banner of Encouragement. After sending e-mails and letters explaining my idea, I received outpourings of sentiment, words of confidence, words of inspiration and words of expectation.   My Seattle women's hiking group gave me a Mount Rainier bandana, their names signed on each of its glaciers and a flag with "Nan" at the top. All the pieces were cool, but they were also big.   By the time I sewed all this wonderful fabric together, adding photos of my mom, kids and grandchildren, the Banner of Encouragement was eight feet long, more than two feet wide and weighed two pounds.   Clearly I did not plan on an extra two pounds in my pack on Kilimanjaro.   A solution would have to present itself.

♪ ♪ ♪ ♪ ♪

My mom, June Berryman Wells, frequently expressed hesitation about this trip.   It had taken her a long time to come to grips with the Parkinson's diagnosis, especially since my dad had died of Lou Gehrig's disease (ALS) in 1972 at age 56.   She tried to convince me, and herself, that this Parkinson's was a product of my imagination; she told me repeatedly the symptoms would go away if I just concentrated on being healthy.   I don't think she could bear the idea of another family member living and dying with a neurodegenerative disease. (Unfortunately, in early 2011 my brother Doug was diagnosed with ALS.   It was impossible to avoid the specter of neurodegenerative disease in our family.)   Consistent with the thinking of her day, she begged me to conserve my energy. During our frequent phone calls the conversation always included, "Don't you think you're doing too much, dear?" "Be careful, dear."   But she knew if I decided to climb Kilimanjaro, I would at least try my best to do it.

We celebrated Mom's ninety-third birthday, April 24, 2011, Easter Sunday, with a family gathering in Traverse City, Michigan, at the home of my oldest brother, Tom Wells.   My daughter, Jodie, came from Seattle with a special birthday gift: Mom's namesake, her great-granddaughter Rosalina June, not quite six months old.

Mom's celebration could not have been more perfect. She was as healthy as could be, excited to meet Rosie, thrilled we all showed up and eager for a party. The day after her birthday we took a walk overlooking the Sleeping Bear dunes. Mom walked half a mile each way, some of it in the sand and some of it on a boardwalk. I loved seeing my ninety-three-year-old Mom so agile and so strong.

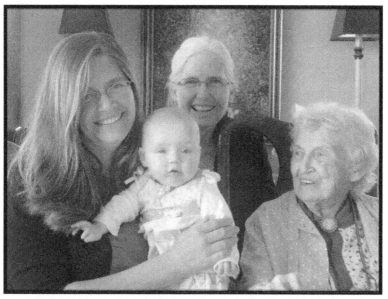

Four generations on Mom's ninety-third birthday

She talked about everything, and nothing, often repeating herself but generally just expressing joy in life and joy for our lives as well. She was so very happy. (I added photo swatches from this event to my Banner of Encouragement.) Although she repeatedly expressed concern about my climbing Mount Kilimanjaro, she promised that no matter what, she would cheer me on until I returned from Africa. We both looked forward to our phone call when I returned.

Exactly five weeks after her Easter birthday, on Sunday May 29, 2011, Mom died. She complained of a stomachache on Thursday. When Tom took her to the doctor, he assured him that a simple operation could resolve her problem. But when the doctor talked to Mom, she had her own ideas. Life had presented increasingly difficult physical and mental challenges. Having watched many friends and acquaintances painfully play the game to the end, she was passionate about not being a burden to others. In addition, she had always been terrified of being kept alive by artificial means, hooked to tubes, unable to walk, living an existence more suitable to the grave than life. She expressed no fear, only confidence that death liberated. For years she had promised to die quickly. We all joked with her

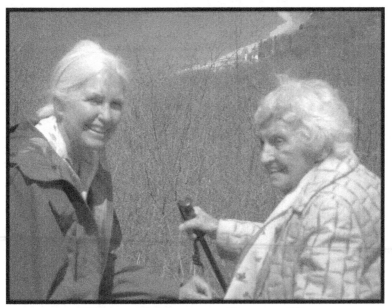

Hiking with Mom near Traverse City

about how timing isn't always a choice. Nonetheless, she insisted she knew how her life would end. She refused the surgery; the next day was her last. She did it her way, as always. Having prepared carefully to climb her mountain, she was more ready than I.

I really couldn't believe she was gone. I felt numb. The trip to Africa lost importance. I wanted to go to Michigan to be with her things, to inhale her fragrance. I wanted to help Tom sort through her belongings, but he was busy and wasn't going to get to it for another few weeks. By then we would be heading for Africa. So I waited to go to Michigan until her memorials in August: a service downstate at her home church in Ferndale, and another up north at our beloved cottage.

I hesitate to write this because it sounds more than a little strange. The day after Mom died, I wrote in my journal:

> "Last night I woke about 3:30 and saw a misty, fog-like figure standing next to Doug's side of the bed. As I pulled myself awake, it disappeared. Later as I was mostly sleeping I could 'hear'/feel Mom calling, 'I'm lost, I'm lost. Help me. I'm lost.' That was most disturbing. I hope she's okay tonight."

Shortly before we left for Africa, I recorded another experience:

> "Last night I had a long talk with Mom. It was after I finally settled down about the trip and relaxed enough to listen. The only time I've heard her before was the night she died, and she was lost and afraid and I comforted her and told her she would find her way. Last night I asked what it was like and she said it was nothing like she thought it would be, but it was good. She is at peace. She's not an entity anymore—hard to say what she is— no talk of reuniting with Dad or family or Jesus—just a general sense of peace. She told me I'll be fine—nothing to worry about at all. I have such a good feeling about her. I'm eager to go to Africa. Even if I walk most of the way alone, I'll be fine. I don't feel alone at all."

Perhaps that conversation is just my mind making up what I wanted to hear, or perhaps it's something else. I don't suppose I'll know until it's my turn.

Before taking off for Africa I climbed thousands more steps with an increasingly heavy pack on my back, and added to my expanding Banner of Encouragement. Shortly after Mom died I began receiving envelopes from her friends in Michigan. More wonderful words of encouragement, words of praise, words of hope, words of confidence. "Be sure your feet are in the right place, then stand firm." "Life is fragile—handle with prayer." and many more. It felt like she was still speaking to me. I proudly sewed swatches from the last letter Mom wrote to me on my Banner of Encouragement, and now I read the messages as I cycle on my trainer in the basement where the Banner hangs on the wall in front of me. I am never alone.

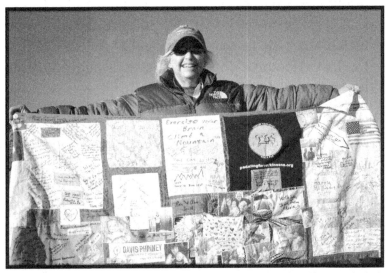

Banner of Encouragement (Photo courtesy of Jeff Rennicke)

ဇ ဇ ဇ ဇ ဇ

The banner became a focal point for our group. In Tanzania we took pictures of it in front of our Arusha Hotel. We took pictures of it at the Machame entrance gate just as we were starting our climb. At key points along the way the banner was brought out and joyfully held high. Despite good intentions, the two pounds quickly became a problem. As much as I had trained, I was still not strong enough to climb with a heavy pack. I could carry it at the lower elevations, meaning from 12,000 to 15,000 feet. But when it came to summit night, although I believed I could climb the mountain, I knew the banner would be more than I could handle. Of course my goal, very much like in the cycling experiences, was to have my supporters close to me. As it turned out, they had to give their encouragement from a few feet away. I needed to carry just bare essentials: food, water, and medication. That night I ruefully passed the banner to our guide. As it turned out, my supporters were close enough.

Parkinson's disease is certainly both mental and physical. Categorized as a movement disorder, it was reflected in my psyche every bit as much or even more than in my physical movement. So many days it was just hard to think, much less to motivate myself to get on the bike. When times were hard, I had my Banner of Encouragement, which represented positive thoughts of people who cared. I promised them all I would do my best. I'm still trying to keep my word.

Chapter 16. Mount Kilimanjaro: The Climb

"I once thought of my mother's stories as history. I thought memory was history. Then I became an historian, and after many years I have come to realize that only careless historians confuse memory and history. *History is the enemy of memory. The two stalk each other across the fields of the past, claiming the same terrain.* History forges weapons from what memory has forgotten or suppressed." [Italics mine]

Richard White, *Remembering Ahanagran*

By researching and telling "the historical truth," historians disrupt memories and restructure the past. My story of climbing Mount Kilimanjaro is based on shaped memories rather than uncovered truth. There is no one "true" story of the Leap of Faith climb. There are as many stories as there are points of view and therefore people who climbed or attempted to climb the mountain, especially on summit night. Each story is valid and each story changes every time it is told as our memories reconstruct our "realities" of the experience.

An historian might be able to sort out sequences of what actually happened on the mountain on summit night, but for those of us who were part of it, each memory is shaped and reshaped as we tell our stories. To some extent, they are all true ... and all false. Perhaps to a greater extent, it doesn't matter.

I know I found meaning in the ascent of Mount Kilimanjaro. Did our effort to stand on top of a mountain actually convey a message of hope and inspiration for other people with neurodegenerative diseases? It's up to them to decide. By doing it, I showed myself that I am capable of much more than I ever thought. RAGBRAI stretched my personal sense of self-efficacy; Kilimanjaro encouraged me to take on tasks I would never have dreamed were within my realm. I realized that, for me, the barriers were not centered in my physical self, however real those barriers brought on by PD were; more than anything they were psychological barriers that gained traction with the disease. Can our climb benefit others? I hope so.

♪ ♪ ♪ ♪ ♪

An entire village supported the climb:

- 131 Tanzanian staff to haul food, water, tents, toilets, our gear bags, four canisters of oxygen and us up the mountain (fifteen were guides);
- Professional photographer, Jeff Rennicke;
- Two American guides, Eric Murphy and Ben Jones from Alpine Ascents International (AAI) in Seattle;
- Parkinson's doctor, Monique Giroux, and physician's assistant, Sierra Farris;
- Organizer, Lori Schneider;
- Nearly fourteen teams of climbers. (One companion left on the first day and two men, one with MS and one with PD, acted as companions for each other, bringing the total group to 25.)

Participants ranged in age from the youngest, a psychologist from Barcelona, age twenty-three, to the oldest, Lori's father/companion, age seventy-nine. Ten climbers, one man and nine women, had varying stages of MS while three younger men and myself had Parkinson's. Our disabilities ranged from barely noticeable to severe. Climbing companions ranged from spouses (Doug and Martha) to friends of Lori and a few who heard about the climb and asked to join. We lived from sea level to high up in the mountains. Most had never climbed a mountain before.

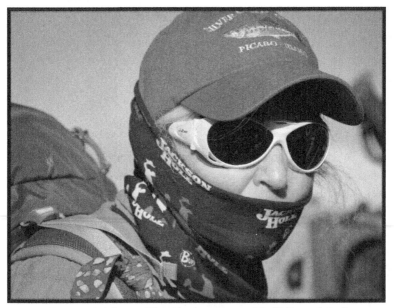

Nan geared up (Photo courtesy of Jeff Rennicke)

We were told to expect to spend five and a half days getting to high camp at 15,500 feet, a long, long night summiting the mountain, and part of the next day returning to a lower camp before leaving Kilimanjaro behind us. Our Machame route (the "Whiskey Route") would allow extra time for acclimation before attempting the summit. I think Machame must mean "harder than the other routes" in Swahili.

As it turned out, this was much more than a walk in the park at high elevation.

Saturday, July 9 Doug and I met John and Martha, Monique and Sierra at Dulles International Airport for the flights to Arusha, Tanzania. Ethiopian Airlines, 11:30 a.m. After a forever plane ride during which Doug nursed the beginnings of a cold, we arrived in Addis Ababa, Ethiopia, at 7:55 a.m., then into Arusha, Tanzania, about 12:15 p.m. on Sunday, July 10.

Because Doug's cold quickly morphed into a bad cough, the six of us went for a town tour with impromptu guides who cheerfully showed us around, found a drugstore and became our new best friends. Although we ostensibly looked for drugs for Doug for two hours, we ended up, after much dodging of vehicles, with a couple of "one-of-a-kind" fabric pictures bought at "deeply reduced" prices. The tour was worth the fee. We crashed about 8:30 p.m. and were up in the night with Doug's worsening cold. I worried about him.

On Monday, July 11, our little group was joined by Micki Babcock, a companion climber, and an "official" guide from the hotel (naturally called Baraka, as were several people we ran into), who was recommended by our guide service, Alpine Ascents International (AAI). We had a more official tour of the town, which replicated what we had done the day before, including the fabric paintings, but which filled out the history of Tanzania in a little more detail. We laughed our way through lunch at Ethiopia Hot and Spicy and learned our first Swahili. I'm *Bebe* (Grandma), Doug is *Babu* (Grandpa). Most of the team arrived rather late Monday night. Instead of taking the advertised town tour, our group spent Tuesday morning on introductions and philosophy, and much of the afternoon checking our gear.

Figuring I could tell him anything important, Doug slept through the introductions but participated in the bag packing/checking exercise. When we introduced ourselves I was particularly intrigued by the prospect of hiking with a MS researcher from the University of Wisconsin, but on the first day of climbing she left without much explanation, leaving eleven companions for the 14 challenged climbers. Monique and Sierra were introduced as our doctor and physician's assistant; Lori, our organizer; and Eric and Ben, our two AAI guides. One of the AAI guides originally assigned to our group had died recently in a tragic fall on Denali, a sobering reminder as to the gravity of the effort we were about to undertake. Ben had been flown in from Everest Base Camp as the emergency backup. Although he had never been to Kilimanjaro, with his strong background of mountain climbing and guiding, he made an excellent addition to the team.

After being declared fit to begin the trek the next day, we optimistically ventured out for our first group dinner, eager to eat and return to the hotel for much needed sleep. Since it was such a large group, it took the restaurant several *hours* to prepare our meals. We wished we had had a three-choice menu or even a buffet. While we waited, acrobats, fire-eaters, and amazing Cirque du Soleil–type entertainers performed, hoping for tips. I would have appreciated them more if I weren't so tired and frustrated. Anxiety exacerbates Parkinson's symptoms and I had ample reason to be anxious. I hated to admit I also had twinges of concern about the organization of this complex undertaking. If we couldn't be fed in the city in a timely way, what would happen when we faced real challenges on the mountain?

The following morning, after yet another review of protocols, we bussed to the entrance of the park to check in for our seven-day adventure, eat a snack and take banner photos. Of the seven climbing routes to ascend Kilimanjaro, the easiest was the Coca-Cola route, the one Lori had taken with her father nineteen years before. Although the Machame route would give us an extra day to acclimate at altitude, we understood it was more difficult than the Coca-Cola route.

For the most part, the group was hopeful, anticipatory. Although many did not exude confidence, as we were nervous about taking on such an unknowable challenge, we bolstered each other's enthusiasm. Most had trained well, and many were outstanding athletes to begin with, not typical multiple sclerosis or Parkinson's patients. All expressed concern as to whether or not we had prepared enough for such an adventure. Many were justifiably worried about how our bodies would react to medications at altitude and how our diseases might present on the mountain.

With great anticipation we signed in and snacked at the entrance gate, took photos and set off to hike the Machame route. Later, as we rounded a bend we saw tables and chairs, even with plastic flowers, and a fancy lunch waiting. I relaxed.

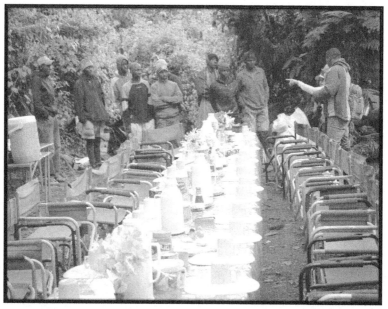

Lunch on the trail (Photo courtesy of Nathan Henwood)

When we arrived at Machame Hut camp (9,500 feet) after dusk, we quickly adopted what would become a daily pattern of finding our gear, selecting a tent from among those that were already in place, arranging our sleeping bags and packs, washing with warm water brought to each tent by the porters, then moving directly to the giant dining tent, a colorful cocoon that seemed to wrap us together each evening. A water-cooler-size bottle of warm water and a bar of soap stationed outside the big tent enabled us to feel relatively sanitized. In addition, we each had our private bottle of hand sanitizer, which we needed little encouragement to use frequently.

After dinner Eric reviewed what we should expect the next day, telling us what to carry in order to be prepared. Then time for chitchat or off to bed, most frequently the latter for us as Doug was battling his cold. Due to his congestion and coughing we slept poorly.

The second day we spent over 10 hours on the trail, including much rock scrambling. Starting at Machame Hut at about 9,500 feet, we crossed the Shira Plateau (12,300 feet) hiking from rain forest to open ground, ended at Shira Hut and camped at Shira Camp (12,500 feet).

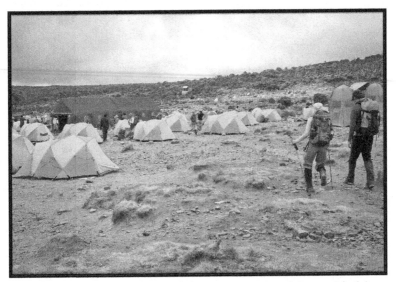

Arriving at Shira Camp (Photo courtesy of Doug Little)

Although the climb was challenging, neither did I find it hard to breathe, nor did I experience any acute mountain sickness like some of my companions. To hopefully ensure that

I continued in good health, I took Diamox—one half of a 125 mg tablet. Other than Doug's congestion and subsequent lack of sleep and energy, life was great.

As we approached each challenge, members of the group supported each other. If one was concerned, another offered encouragement. At one point I came into a rest stop with a debilitating pain in my shoulder that nearly brought me to tears. Stephanie, a physical therapist with MS, immediately leaped through a boulder field to get to me and within moments relieved the pain.

Later she entertained the group with a portable hula hoop she had packed with her. Imagine hula hooping at over 12,000 feet! (Or having the determination to carry one with her.) Sean made a hilarious video of sixty-five-year-old me hula hooping at Shira Camp much to the astonishment of those who did not know that, to a child of the 50s, twirling a hula hoop was as easy as riding a bike.

Although I had to meet personal challenges, I never felt alone. In nearly all situations, I felt I was part of a team. Along easier stretches and at rest breaks we talked about our lives, our difficulties, what strategies we had developed for facing challenges and how people intended to change their attitudes and behaviors after this experience. As a resident female elder, I generally listened to the conversations rather than taking a lead. Most of the other women could have been my daughters or even granddaughters. Some people had energy to talk with each other as they relaxed at the end of each climbing day. Others of us were exhausted and tried to get as much rest as possible. Those who were sick did their best to hide their illnesses, tough to do when coughing or vomiting. We saw each other's variations on Parkinson's and MS and just how each disease fit the "designer" description.

A key to our cohesiveness was that, even though during the day we were strung out over the mountain, we could still see each other, plus we gathered at regular intervals to rest and eat. Some hikers were clearly stronger than others, but I felt no sense of competition or isolation—until summit night and the days after.

Doug was still coughing badly and sleeping poorly. The third day on the trail was another long day with the option to hike an extra loop to the Lava Tower, over 15,000 feet. I wanted to go to Lava Tower in part just to see if I could do it. Friends from Seattle who had made the trip said it really was worth the extra loop. Doug assured me he would be fine if I left him, and he was. Although I spent most of my time trying to keep up with the others, I relished my moment of independence.

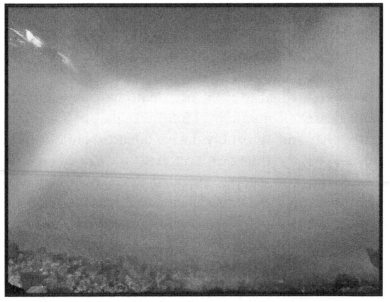

White Rainbow (Fog Bow) on the trail into Barranco
(Photo by Doug Little)

Independence aside, the detour to Lava Tower made me come to grips with how much I relied on Doug for even the smallest decisions. Some indecision is just my nature. However, with Parkinson's it became more and more difficult to force myself to decide anything. On the Lava Tower hike when I developed a little blister on my toe, Ben stopped right away to make sure it was properly cared for, pointing out that a little problem early on would probably cause a lot of pain later. Not wanting to be a bother, I had walked quite a ways before deciding to mention the blister to him.

To acclimate to the elevation we climbed up and down, finally dropping down to reach the campsite: 12,800 feet at the base of the Great Barranco Wall. As we entered the campsite, a thick mist prevented our seeing what lay in store for the next day. We heard it was a steep climb, not a technical rock climb, but it would take sustained effort to make the scramble.

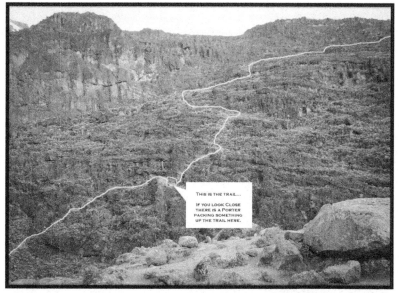

Trail up the Great Barranco Wall
(Photo courtesy of Nathan Henwood)

The hike on Saturday, the fourth day, was short but vertical. When we awoke, the dense mist had lifted and the obvious challenge lay before us. We shuddered as we watched heavily laden porters inching their way up the rock face, all too aware we would not be far behind. A source of constant amazement was watching the porters carry bulky weights on their backs and their heads, sometimes up to 100 pounds each. While we dragged our sorry selves up the rocks in our state-of-the-art climbing apparel and formfitting boots, they scrambled past in their ill-fitting shoes or sandals, carrying four times the weight we bore.

The Great Barranco Wall put to rest any idea that this was a ramble in a park at elevation. Much of the time we gripped sharp rocks with three points—white-knuckled fingers or curled, cramped toes—to make sure we did not fall. Each person carefully helped the next person understand exactly where the foot and hand placements must be. Some voices carried an edge of terror.

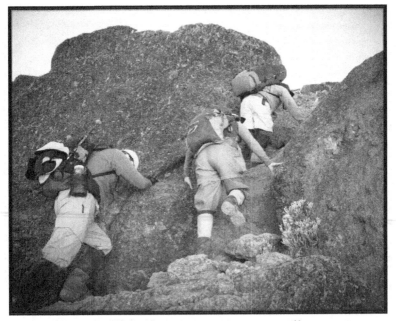

Scaling the Great Barranco Wall
(Photo courtesy of Nathan Henwood)

The guides anticipated our needs and provided for us. Whether it was a timely hand on the elbow, singing encouragement, or taking the poles or the pack when the going became increasingly steep or treacherous, they knew what needed to be done and did not hesitate to do it. We scaled the Great Barranco Wall, feeling justifiably proud of our accomplishments: individual firsts for all but a very few, certainly a first for me. Like Potter's Hill on RAGBRAI, it wasn't something I wanted to do again.

We descended from our high point of 14,500 feet to the lower elevation of Karanga River Camp at about 13,000 feet. Although we had come a long way, I felt intimidated realizing we had another mile of elevation gain before we would stand atop Kilimanjaro.

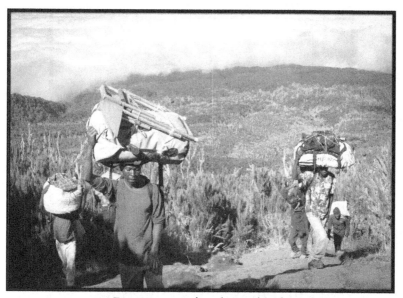

Porters carrying large loads
(Photo courtesy of Nathan Henwood)

Doug continued to have a tough time with congestion, causing me to be concerned about his summit attempt. Eric had told us repeatedly that if he saw people in trouble he would tell them to return to the Kosovo high camp, and we were to trust his judgment.

One woman had not held down any food for four days straight. Several others, including our medical staff of Monique and Sierra, suffered from altitude headaches severe enough that they often did not come to dinner but went straight to their tents to try to ease the pain and rest as best they could. Another young woman, so compromised by her MS she could hardly hike at all, gamely plugged along. I didn't recall any exclusion criteria when we signed up, such as level of disability, history of acute mountain sickness, asthma or IBS. Some things, such as the vomiting and cough, could not be predicted.

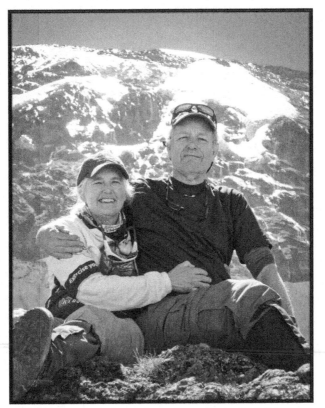

Brief respite (Photo by Doug Little)

Every evening Eric or Ben used a device called a pulse oximeter, or pulse-ox, to measure our pulse rate and the level of oxygen in our blood. At sea level, a person is at risk if their blood oxygen level is below 90 percent. At high altitude one can function at that level, but obviously it becomes increasingly difficult and at some point dangerous to continue to climb with too little oxygen in the blood. A few in the group had readings in the high 60s or low 70s. Others of us were in the 90s. I felt certain that Eric would err on the side of safety and not allow those with low numbers to attempt the summit. I took comfort in my erroneous assumption.

Sunday, July 17 we hiked six or seven hours (a "short hike," as Eric would usually say, sort of jokingly) to our high camp at Kosovo. First we headed to Barafu (appropriately sounds like Barf You) (14,650 feet), the quite literally garbage-covered intersection of various trails, where we merged with ever-increasing numbers of teams of people, all intending to stand on the roof of Africa that night. We quickly ate lunch and gratefully pushed on to Kosovo, our high camp at 15,600 feet. When we neared the high camp, the porters repeatedly returned to the last flowing water to bring back container after container to meet our eating and washing needs. Each container was the equivalent of an office water-cooler bottle.

At Kosovo we learned how the night would unfold. Eric had us select which of three groups we wanted to hike in: A Group, the slowest, would leave first, followed by B and C at 15 minute intervals. When he told us to self-select our groups, nearly everyone, including Doug and I, chose group B.

I had trusted that by this time Eric would know each of us well enough to assign us to our groups, so I was surprised when he had us self-select and allowed everyone to go. As he had been tracking our blood oxygen levels every day, I expected those measurements would affect his decisions to allow individuals to continue to climb the mountain. Doug's congestion was no better and his pulse ox reading hovered between 68 and 73 percent whereas mine was consistently 89 to 92. Some people had low blood oxygen levels, while others had suffered for days from headaches, nausea, and indigestion consistent with acute mountain sickness; but individuals were neither advised to nor denied the opportunity to climb. Everyone decided to try. I wondered why Eric, an experienced mountain guide, was leaving potentially life-and-death decisions up to novice climbers, some of whom were already compromised when we began to climb Kilimanjaro and even more compromised by the time we were to attempt the summit ascent. I thought perhaps I was just being unduly anxious. He proved worthy of our trust.

More concerned about Doug's health than whether or not he stood at the top of the mountain, I asked him if he thought he should go. He let me know later he did not appreciate my suggestion. I never thought about it as an issue of confidence; it seemed to me the measurable risk was unreasonably high. More anxiety. I think of that point as the beginning of my confusion about what happened over the next few days.

After being given our different wake-up times and already oxygen deprived, we slowly slid into our tents and very carefully packed our gear for summit night, quite literally weighing what we felt necessary to carry. For about three hours we tried to sleep, but it was generally impossible.

Summit Night

At 10:00 p.m., dressed and fortified with porridge, we anxiously awaited permission to begin the climb. Group A left shortly before the large group B. Most difficult to bear, the bitter 15 degree cold chilled me through and through, in spite of all my gear and hand warmers. As we milled around, waiting, a huge full moon eerily lighted Kilimanjaro, strangely suspended between a cloud bank below us and the clear sky above, a surreal night. Lights crawled ahead of us up the mountain, like a giant centipede inching its way to the top. Finally our group struck out at about 10:45 p.m., joining that centipede of headlamps inching its way up the mountain. As we stepped onto the trail, Doug whispered to me, "I know you can make it." I nodded.

People moved at their own pace, most semblance of "companion climbers" discarded as individuals hunkered in to their own mental and physical spaces. Attempting to keep some sense of the "plan", our B group broke into smaller parts, overtook A and blended the two, with some small groups moving forward more quickly while others lagged. Doug and I lagged. Group C quickly threaded its way through all of us, along with strangers from other teams.

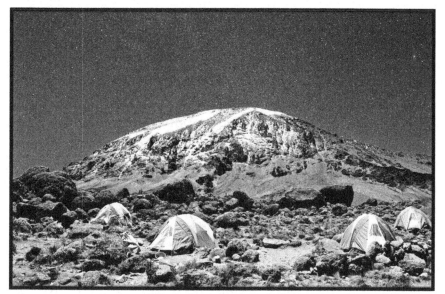

Kilimanjaro by Moonlight
(Photo courtesy of Jeff Rennicke)

Doug's cold, his low blood oxygen level and his incessant cough slowed him significantly. We stayed together. The young woman with the most severe MS and her companion were barely moving. Finally she said she was falling asleep and was afraid she would fall over and knock someone off the mountain. She had to go down. Her companion descended with her. Instead of moving on at our own pace, the few of us who had been hiking together waited a long time in the bitter, windy cold, about 20 minutes, possibly more, for our Tanzanian guide to find Eric and then for him to arrange their descent. As we stood still and the temperature continued to drop, I thought the end of my thumb had frostbite. I couldn't feel my fingertips no matter what warm-up exercises I tried.

We shuffled slowly after the first two headed down. Breathing hard to take in oxygen and coughing constantly, Doug finally said he had to quit. He told me afterwards he was taking three breaths for each step. Increasingly fearful, giving in to anxiety, I convinced myself he might be spitting up blood, although he said he was not. As we waited again for Eric, I could feel the chill move deeper into every part of my body. Eric told me later he was afraid to tell Doug to go down because he respected his decision-making powers so profoundly.

On my own, half frozen, I continued, knowing I needed to move more quickly to warm up but unable to do so. I was freezing and slow. I just kept going, hoping for the best. People kept either passing or dropping back. It was horrible . . . and wonderful. Although the scene was beautiful—dreamlike, with the full moon and a few stars—I was cold, so cold, I felt the night would never end. We kept walking ever so slowly. At one point we passed a team member who was really sick and eventually descended for oxygen (needing to tell other hikers how to operate the tank since no one with medical training was at high camp); another time we joined a small group watching two strangers from another climbing team who had collapsed. Our Tanzanian guide made us wait in case he was supposed to help. I had no idea what he could do to help and he didn't seem to know either.

If we waited much longer, I knew I would be the next one escorted down, so I told him I was just going to continue, whether he joined me or not. The other women from our cadre agreed. Our guide stayed with us. Connie, an authentic mountaineer, scampered to join us after her companion who needed the oxygen started the descent. I was too slow for 67 year-old Connie, who forged ahead. I continued, sometimes picking up or dropping people from our team as I struggled up the rocks. So focused on my own ascent, I only recognized that others were with me if they were in my immediate field of focus. If they hiked ahead or dropped behind, it was as if they had never been with me. I do recall that Ines, the young psychologist from Barcelona, accompanied me a long time.

Affected by the double whammy of Parkinson's and cold, my fingers refused to work. Since I couldn't manipulate my food wrappers, the little chunks of GU Energy Gel and Clif SHOT BLOKS were accessible only by asking the guide to go into my pack, find them, unwrap them and stick them in my mouth. I generally had four bites of energy at a time. The water in the bottles inside my pack was so nearly frozen that it was more effort than reward to get a drink. Our guide gave me sips now and then as if I were a baby, but only when I asked for it, which wasn't nearly often enough. Although I became more and more dehydrated, I was oblivious to my body's need.

On we struggled, eventually joined by Lori, who had had to send her father down, each of his arms draped over a guide's shoulder. As all this time I didn't know how Doug was doing, I worried whenever my thoughts moved out of my mental fog and turned to him. At that point, Parkinson's or not, I didn't need extra anxiety.

At some point the other women went ahead leaving Ines to stay with me as long as she could. Finally, as I was just resting so often or going so slowly, she asked my permission and moved forward. I still feel utterly grateful to her for keeping me company for so long, even though we seldom spoke.

On our several encounters as he raced up and down the trail, Eric encouraged me to hustle, but I was nearly frozen and couldn't climb as steadily as he wanted me to: 45 to 60 minutes without a break. I was fortunate if I went 45 to 60 steps without a break and seldom made it even that far. When I encountered him, shirt open, chest covered with sweat while I was so cold I could barely move, I realized I had never seen a person under such stress. His dedication to those most severely challenged in the group was heroic. Later he told me he ascended the mountain five times that night. He both tended to climbers scattered along the trail and returned to the Kosovo high camp to check that early returnees who were helping each other as best they could were safe enough to be left on their own.

I followed a guide, probably Joachim, staring at his boots and occasionally thinking how hard it must be for him to go so slowly. Not looking happy, he kept glancing back to see if I still moved. I recall asking him to sing, but he never sang.

I never got a headache or nausea–just cold and tired beyond words. I thought about words on the banner, Doug, Mom, but mostly I didn't think, although I tried to focus on something tangible. Sometimes I counted. I looked up the mountain, recited names on the banner, counted again, sang snatches of "The Impossible Dream" in my head, never the whole song, and concentrated on breathing and keeping moving forward and up. I recall watching myself put my foot on a rock and go up, thinking, "Look what you did! Your leg went over that rock!" From somewhere out of my body I watched my progress up the mountain. Sometimes I felt like I was asleep, but I kept walking, following lights and the path. I was so alone . . . and so not alone.

Breathe, breathe, breathe, *step.* Breathe, breathe, breathe, *step.* Breathe, breathe, breathe, *step.* Breathe, breathe, breathe, *step.* Ahead of me the headlamps and the full moon continued to light my way through the night up Mount Kilimanjaro.

At 3:00 a.m., dawn was a long way off. Although people were around me, I was only vaguely aware of them, focusing instead on whatever internal resources I could muster. Like thoughts of family. Again and again my mind drifted to my great grandfather, Henry Byron Wells. During the Alaska gold rush in 1898 he made the arduous journey from Skagway to Dawson City and found a little gold. In January he developed dysentery and was told he would surely die and be stacked like cordwood with other winter corpses, waiting for the spring thaw to be buried.

Life is about choices. Henry Byron decided if he were going to end up dead in a snow bank, he might as well expire while trying to get home. I had read in an old newspaper that he had packed enough supplies for thirty days in his primitive pack. Twenty-eight days later he walked into Skagway. As I slogged slowly up Mount Kilimanjaro, my mind reflected on the fortitude and strength it had taken to walk through the Alaskan cold and dark—with no headlamp and no sunrise to anticipate. If he could take a step, I could take a step. It's not surprising I was thinking of death and survival that night on the mountain.

My journey from high camp to the summit and back to high camp would be, after all, less than 14 hours, not 28 days, and I wasn't even sick, just weighed down with disease. I was also nearly sixty-six-years-old and a woman, and if not the oldest, surely one of few senior women with Parkinson's to climb Mount Kilimanjaro. Other issues aside, as I wound my way up the mountain that night I knew that if I kept my focus, I would make it to the top and back. Doug believed in me: he said he knew I could do it, and I knew I could too.

Eric told us our back-up goal was to make it at least to the false summit—Stella Point, an hour from the true summit—by the time the sun rose, but our primary goal was to see the sunrise from the top of Kilimanjaro. He firmly told us that if we didn't reach Stella Point by 10:30, we would have to turn around. When the sky started to color around 6:00 a.m., I wasn't anywhere near either goal. But as I felt the first warm rays of sun an hour before I reached Stella Point, hardly on track to meet the sunrise goal, I didn't really care about rules and timelines. The sun on the horizon meant that eventually it would get much warmer. I knew I could get there if I just kept to the *pole pole* pattern (poh-lay poh-lay, Swahili for slowly, slowly). One step at a time, pole, pole. As though on autopilot, I moved in a foggy zone, aware I was within Eric's time constraint, defining my own goals. I wouldn't possibly quit when I was so close.

I had heard somewhere that the coldest part of the night is the hour before dawn. I so wished for dawn. I begged for dawn. When the sun rose long before I reached the false summit, with its rays came a little warmth and the knowledge that I most certainly would complete this climb. Finally my guide and I stepped over the rim. I wept, and weep again just thinking of it. The pre-climb literature had advertised that someone would be there with hot tea or coffee, but there was neither person nor coffee when we arrived. I recall being confused, as I had been looking forward optimistically, if not realistically, to both.

Joachim and I headed along the rim walk for another hour to reach the actual summit. With clear skies and clouds below us, we could see forever. This was the roof of Africa! Along the graveled path we passed members of our group, most of whom were sick, dizzy, nauseous, or complaining of massive headaches but utterly joyful they had stood on top of Kilimanjaro. We shared many hugs, and lots of concern as to how they were really doing. It took another hour to reach the top from Stella Point, another 600-foot elevation gain, which seemed like nothing after hiking through the steep scree. During this whole experience, I never had any sign of acute mountain sickness unless my out of body sensations count. I don't know if I could have walked all night with a headache or nausea as many others did.

I hugged Nathan, who was staggering and babbling uncontrollably, his Parkinson's medicines clearly not working. Monique and Sierra looked pretty out of it, but they were on their feet. I hugged some others and quickly continued on.

The Summit

After an hour or so of relatively flat walking, on Monday morning, July 18 I moved briskly to the summit sign which was already flanked by Connie, Ines and Lori. We made some banner videos and cried tears of exhaustion and relief, with some incredulity for good measure.

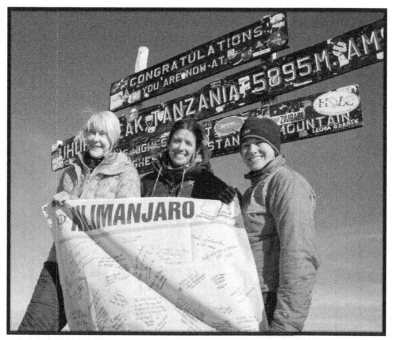

Three strong women, two with MS
(Photo courtesy of Jeff Rennicke)

I was happy to be there, and I was crying, choking with emotion and exhaustion. On the video I asked Eric to make, I expressed gratitude to those who had helped get me there: people in our group and people on the banner. I felt relief I had been able to follow through and complete this challenge—underscored with inexpressible relief it was over. At that moment I didn't think about Doug or Mom or anything other than what was exactly in front of me. I felt safe in the sunshine—in the warming light—not alone.

We were seven at the top. Jeff, our professional photographer asked to leave, as he had been at the summit since before dawn and was utterly exhausted. He had photographed nearly everyone in the group who had summited but me; his camera equipment was stowed and he had neither the energy nor desire to get it out again. I didn't blame him, but I couldn't deny it made me feel like a disconnected burden, a loose end. I wanted him to take my photo as he had everyone else's. Not to be. Lori used her camera as Doug had ours in his pocket. We made a little Flip video of the banner and the summit sign, and Eric made a video too. Because I asked, Jeff stayed just long enough to be in my video; then he was off. Photography session over, the women left while I slowly directed my hands to pack my camera and my banner.

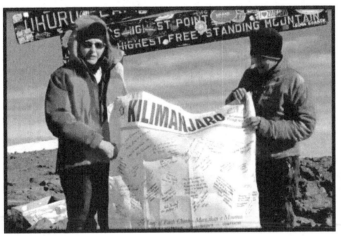

Nan and Lori at the summit of Mount Kilimanjaro

Eric, Joachim and I stood alone. Quiet. Unbelievably quiet. No worries, no sound—just the wind. Relatively warm. I was surprised at the grimy landscape nearly barren of snow or ice. It was strangely beautiful in the sunshine, some glaciers sparkling, a lake in the crater—a marker on a glacier outside of the cone showing how much that glacier had melted. It did not appear the ice would last long.

I wanted to stay to absorb the experience and just be still, but Eric prodded me to leave. I stood on the roof of Africa for about 15 minutes.

I reluctantly left for the hour's walk back to Stella Point, Eric at my side, Joachim following dutifully. When he saw I could walk pretty fast, Eric commented on my speed and, assured I was fine, trotted off to catch the others. Like a good shepherd, Eric made sure the last sheep would make it back to the fold before checking on the others.

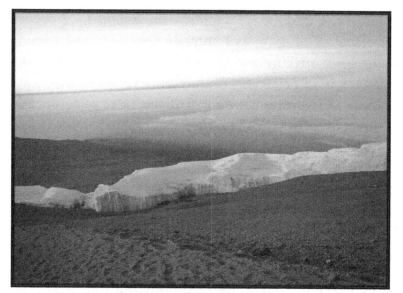

Glacier on the roof of Africa
(Photo courtesy of Nathan Henwood)

At Stella Point I realized I had not taken my PD medicine, so I took it at 9:52 a.m., about 11 hours after we had left high camp. I was three hours late taking it, setting me up for the massive, uncontrolled tremors that occurred later in the day. I still couldn't undo the clips on my pack or open the water bottle, so Joachim helped me. I was the last of our group up there. Actually, Joachim and I were the last of any group that day.

Shortly after starting a scree hop down, on our right we could see our high camp tents and, on the trail, Lori, Connie and Ines who had gone ahead. For whatever reason, Joachim headed left, despite my protestations. He didn't seem to know the way down! As we moved further and further away from the camp, my frustration increased. After what seemed an eternity we came upon a group of guides hunting for stragglers.

Delighted to be going the right way, I rabbit hopped through scree, much to the astonishment of the guides who wanted to hold my elbows to keep me from falling. Inexplicably, I had no problems with balance. I turned my watch off at 12:32 p.m. as I entered Kosovo high camp, nearly 14 hours after striking out for the summit and possibly over an hour longer than necessary finding our way back. Indicative of my intense dehydration, I had urinated only once during that entire time, and that was when we were nearly to the bottom.

Doug and a cook were waiting. Doug had been standing there for hours, scanning the mountain for a familiar red parka. He nearly broke my ribs with his hugs. I buried my head in his chest, eager for him to take charge. He thanked the Tanzanian guides for getting me down. I never had been so exhausted in my life, so exhausted I couldn't even feel happy I had done it. I believe I almost didn't register it was over. Doug told me I would make it and I did. Perhaps it would mean more to me later on. At that point, it was just the hardest thing I had ever done and I was numbingly grateful it was over.

As I stumbled toward our tent, a couple of people stepped forward to congratulate me for making it to the top. I couldn't even talk to them. I could barely walk, much less respond intelligently. I think I just stared at them. I wondered where everyone was. Why wasn't this like RAGBRAI, teammates cheering for the last person to arrive? I know I expected something else, an esprit de corps like I had experienced while cycling, something to fold me into the group again, but except for Doug, I was essentially alone. I was too exhausted to do more than mentally register the difference. Although it was a far cry from RAGBRAI, quite possibly the others were nearly as exhausted as I, unable to cheer.

I vaguely recall attempting to eat something before packing my gear with Doug and taking off for the next lower campsite. Exhausted, I couldn't get much food in my mouth. I was hungry, but between my Parkinson's tremor and my frail state I was shaking so hard I could not hold the spoon or even hold the edges of the bowl to just drink my meal. My hands shook wildly like a drummer performing a solo. Even though I had clearly moved past a physical limit, I carried on because there was just no other choice.

With few people left at Kosovo, we started to the next lower camp, another long walk, made a little easier by the increase in oxygen and harder by the slippery logs, sharp rocks and mud on the trail. I remember thinking I was doing well and hearing later I was so clumsy I was exceedingly funny. The descent took five and a half hours, with two guides and Doug helping me to stand upright. We finally arrived at the lower elevation camp at 12,000 plus feet, ate dinner and collapsed. Those who had summited quickly held court, telling jokes and stories, laughing and drinking beer, reliving their climb, especially noting how relatively easy it was for them. Listening to them, I realized that, unlike at RAGBRAI, I did not belong. This had nothing to do with PD or MS; we were individuals reacting as the real people we were before diagnosis and we continued to be in spite of neuro-degenerated or healthy brains.

We walked out the next day. The woman who was afraid she would fall asleep and knock someone off the mountain was carried down to a road in a cart. She said the ride was so painful it would have been better if she had been shot before starting down.

Eventually Lori's dad was driven out. The truck that came for him picked us up on the way back. I wished they had picked us up on their way to fetch him. We slogged along a muddy road from hell for about four hours; it likely would have been seven if the truck hadn't picked us up. When we arrived at the gate, the celebration lunch was nearly over; we faced empty serving bowls instead of the advertised feast. Again, we had missed all the congratulatory/celebratory events except for the locals swarming around trying to sell trinkets. Still exhausted, confused and suffocating from the noise, I was eager to leave. Later I heard there had been music and dancing and a delightful celebration and luncheon before we arrived. But, because I moved so slowly, we missed it all.

Summiting defined the great divide. At one point a woman crowed that everyone on the PD team made it to the top. Standing next to her, Doug asked whose team he was on. She became flustered and answered that she just meant those with PD. As Lori had repeatedly emphasized the importance of the effort we were *all* making, some apparently had heard a different message than I.

After we returned to the Arusha hotel, washed our hair and ourselves and enjoyed putting on clean clothes, we gathered for dinner. I sensed an almost tangible tension between people who had summited the mountain easily and those who had had to turn back or who had had a hard time of it. Once again, the successful climbers regaled each other with their stories, but did not ask about the others' experiences.

It took a long time for me to realize that this was a positive response to our illnesses. None of us was being judged or coddled based on our failing brains. For that moment in time we all sat squarely on the same page and, just like in real life, some won and some lost. The winners celebrated and the losers endured the celebration, just like normal people do.

After the Climb

The trek up Kilimanjaro was followed by three exciting days of safaris in national parks and an early morning balloon ride over the Serengeti that ended with a champagne breakfast under an acacia tree. Instead of scrambling over rocks, we enjoyed hanging onto truck seats as we bounced over rutted roads in high energy searches for wild animals. Once again, we easily could have been part of a National Geographic special.

On our final morning in the Serengeti we loaded into four tour trucks headed for the balloon ride. I eagerly anticipated "a romantic leisurely float on warm air currents, sun rising slowly over the Serengeti, a world of wildlife below." As it turned out, getting to the balloon was anything but romantic. All four trucks took off in the inky black night, racing through the canopy of foliage.

Soon into the ride down the rutted road, branches swishing against the vehicle, our truck, the last in line, stalled in lion country. We sat, listening to the sounds of the awakening jungle, sadly convinced the final event would be a story we heard from others. As only a brief window of opportunity existed for us to get into the balloon baskets and rise before the air currents shut down the operation, each minute that ticked

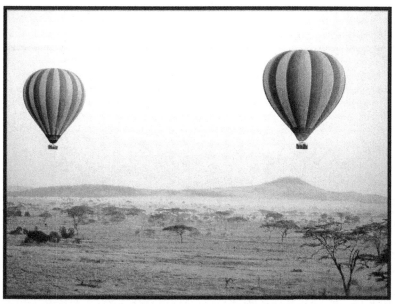

Floating over the Serengetti
(Photo by Doug Little)

away decreased our chances. Finally the hotel switchboard opened, and another driver raced to our rescue. Although it seemed impossible to make up the half hour we had lost watching and listening to the jungle emerging from the night, our driver determined to do his best.

When we arrived at the site, other balloons already aloft, people screamed at us to run. Nearly missing the opportunity, I was tossed in the basket like a bag of grain. Another story. For the next hour we floated over the Serengeti, silences broken by squeals of delight and the whoosh of burners going on to make us rise to miss trees or to pursue elephants, giraffes, hippos, lions, the wildlife of the Serengeti racing below us. Magical!

Too soon, we saw a lone acacia tree surrounded by tables draped with white linens and waiters standing at attention with trays of champagne. Floating over the Serengeti, I was so removed from that night on the mountain, from the cold, from the weariness, from the concern, from the anxiety and challenge of testing my own depths of physical and emotional reserves, it almost felt as though I hadn't climbed the mountain.

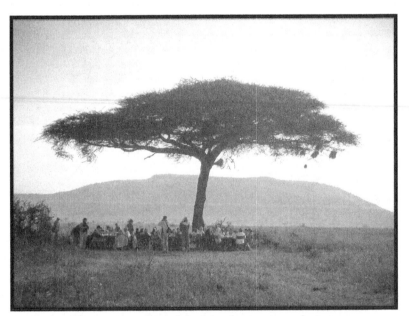

Champagne breakfast under an acacia tree
(Photo by Doug Little)

I still felt separated from the group in intangible ways, eager to return to my own life, to focus on family and wellness rather than competition.

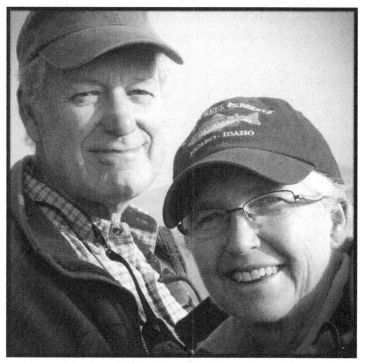

Together

Last night in Africa

On our last night in Arusha, three of the women with MS, two companion climbers, and Doug and I spent hours over dinner attempting to sort out what opportunity this trip presented in the grand scheme of our lives and our diseases. No obvious answers emerged. Lori had designed this trip *"to help others with a neurodegenerative disease regain their emotional strength and to give hope to those on the team and others that they can still pursue dreams in their own life."* (From the Empowerment Through Adventure website.)

Did our experiences bear this out? That remained to be seen. It was self-evident that if any tragedy had happened to one of the challenged climbers on the Kilimanjaro Leap of Faith, Lori's message of empowerment would have been lost. Whereas our trip showed that *some* individuals *might* move beyond perceived limitations, it did not prove or even suggest that most people with neurodegenerative diseases would be able to do so. Hopefully our experience would at least encourage others to try.

We left the Arusha Hotel at 1:30 a.m. on July 24, on what was to be my brother Doug's last birthday. We flew from Arusha to Addis Ababa, to Rome, to Washington, DC, and finally to Seattle.

Home July 25, 2011, 3:25 p.m.

Reflections

I do not believe people can do anything we set our minds to. Obviously we have various physical, mental and financial resources as well as other commitments of time and energy. Unfortunately, some people are not able to cycle to mitigate their PD symptoms. Whereas the big climb, the big event, grabs attention, for most individuals setting short-term, attainable goals is more productive than making the dramatic gesture that may cause permanent damage or accelerate the disease's progression in the long run. However, the big inspirational event undeniably has its place as something for people to point to and say, "If she can do that, surely I can do something for myself as well."

People with Parkinson's can and should be empowered. We neither need to curl up and bemoan our diagnosis nor prove to anyone that we won't let our disease slow us down. Parkinson's will slow us down. Although perhaps we can be in control of our lives more than we are led to believe, the truth is we have a progressive neurodegenerative disease that might be mitigated but won't be cured by medicine, exercise or belief systems. We are in complete charge of our attitudes, but only to some limited extent, our disease.

By the end of July 2011, my PD symptoms had returned, intensified with cramps, instability and gait issues. Most unsettling, I regressed cognitively. I resumed cycling, hoping to at least return to where I was prior to the trip. I got part way there, both physically and cognitively. Although Kilimanjaro exacted a personal toll, I believe the toll was worth it for me.

Cycling is not for everyone. However, if 10 percent of PD patients can mitigate their symptoms, that's 100,000 out of an estimated 1,000,000 PD patients in the United States alone. I would be happy with that. People with Parkinson's don't have to climb Mount Kilimanjaro to be empowered. Thousands can just get on a bike or do other intense aerobic exercises to experience some freedom from some symptoms. It is surely worth a try.

🏔 🏔 🏔 🏔 🏔

There is a certain mystique to climbing Mount Kilimanjaro. People tell me they are inspired by the fact that I made the trip and actually reached the summit at age sixty-five, coping with Parkinson's every step of the way. At the time, I felt anything but inspirational; I felt astonishingly tired, more tired and cold than I ever thought I could be. It was the hardest thing I've ever done and the hardest thing I ever hope to do.

What possessed me to make this trip in the first place? As strange as it sounds, I went because I was asked. I was honored that someone thought I could do it. Although I had done plenty of hiking, I had never climbed a mountain, so this was a new experience and challenge for me, one Doug and I could do together. Our bucket list had already changed because of Parkinson's, so why not add this new challenge? Sierra had told me I was invited "because [I] kicked butt riding across Iowa."

I rode my bike across Iowa the first time because Jay Alberts invited me. I rode across Iowa again and again because

I enjoyed the people and it was fun and we were raising money for PFP, the organization that had made such a profound impact on my life. When I was first asked about climbing Mount Kilimanjaro, there was talk of making a video, or raising funds for MS and Parkinson's research, or in some way using the trip to advance knowledge and understanding of the diseases. Although none of those things was in place when we left for Africa, the important outcome is that the trip has made a positive impact on those who participated and others who have heard about it.

Why did I keep climbing when Doug turned back? I had thought the plan for the climb was for each challenged individual to have a healthy companion to watch out for them. I realized shortly into the summit climb that I was mistaken; climbing Mount Kilimanjaro was essentially a personal mission. Even Lori kept climbing after her father had to return to high camp. I can recall only one companion who descended with her partner. Doug told me he knew I could do it and I believed myself I could do it. With that in mind, barring any insurmountable barrier, I would do my best to summit.

Was I in as much danger as I thought I was? Yes, I think so. Climbing Mount Kilimanjaro was not a romantic enterprise. Although the trip was interesting, educational and many times fun, for me summit night was grueling. I'm thankful I didn't have to make any critical decisions that night as I doubt that all my cylinders were firing. Kilimanjaro is 19,340 feet high. People occasionally die on Mount Kilimanjaro. It's fortunate none of us did.

Stepping back from my pain of the moment, there emerges a message of hope and inspiration for people with Parkinson's and other neurodegenerative diseases. Many people have told me that this effort has inspired them to think of themselves differently even though they have PD. If I have inspired another to take that important step—to think of *self* as more or other than *patient*—then my efforts have been worthwhile. I trained for months and completed a most challenging task, but the climb up and down took one week. Dramatic as that week was, it does not compare with the long haul of living day by day with the disease. Every day of our lives—every day—we struggle to get up, go to swimming or dance or tai chi or whatever we do to get past our barriers. We struggle to ensure there is meaning in our lives. Every day, we PwPs climb a mountain higher than Mount Kilimanjaro—and no one is there to cheer.

To me, this message is fundamentally different from one that claims you can do anything if you only put your mind to it. Some say PD must not be allowed to be an impediment to achieving life goals. I know PD is a major barrier for me and for everyone I've met who has the disease, and I know its inexorable direction: facing higher barriers with increasingly diminished capacity to surmount them. Parkinson's accelerates the subtractions of aging.

When a person is told she can succeed if she only tries hard enough, there is an implicit underlying statement that if she does not succeed, she has not tried hard enough and somehow the failure rests in her, not in the course of the disease or something completely external. She is guilty if she fails. We have enough problems without adding guilt to the mixture. Stretching our goals is healthy. Beating ourselves up is not.

When people look at me, a little white-haired lady, spinning on her bicycle as she talks about Parkinson's, climbing mountains and riding her bike across Iowa, many are inspired to get up out of their chairs and walk around the block. My goal is to help others define and achieve their goals. That is the hope and inspiration I try to share with others from climbing Mount Kilimanjaro.

Chapter 17. Making Pedaling For Parkinson's Sustainable

The first of many Pedaling For Parkinson's programs opened at the Mill Creek YMCA just north of Seattle shortly after we returned from Kilimanjaro. After encountering so many difficulties establishing a PFP program the year before, I had despaired. We had four tandem bikes and no place to go. Partnering with a hospital had presented bureaucratic and logistical barriers. PwPs definitely wanted to participate in such a program; they needed an opportunity. Where to find a confluence of bicycles, trained staff, a commitment to healthy living and open minds? The YMCA, of course!

🚲 🚲 🚲 🚲 🚲

First, some background information to explain how this serendipitous partnership came about. I graduated from college when I was twenty-one and began teaching junior high English that fall of 1967 in a suburb of Detroit. Bored with my social life, I begged my law student brother Bob to please set me up on a blind date for a weekend. Doug Little, brother Bob's co-worker in the law school cafeteria at the University of Michigan Law School, agreed to commit for one night of a weekend. (Later I heard he didn't want to get stuck for two nights.) After four extended dates, Doug and I were married and moved to Philadelphia, where I taught English and he worked for the Pennsylvania Crime Commission as a special agent. Later, with law school finally behind us, we moved to Seattle, had kids and I volunteered. Prosaic story thus far.

When I decided to return to paid work, I had four jobs in one year, eventually landing as Director of International

Programs at Metrocenter YMCA, a creative think tank within the Seattle YMCA. (I applied because I liked the job title, not because I knew anything about international programs.)

The Seattle YMCA was home to both Metrocenter, directed by Jennifer Parker, and the YMCA of the USA Office for Asia, headed by Bill Sieverling. Bill and Jennifer decided the YMCA needed a new, international youth leadership program based on education and the environment. They selected me to be the director of the new YMCA Earth Corps, which has grown into a tremendously successful endeavor.

In 1991 Bill arranged for me to guide a three-week trip for fifteen youths to Hong Kong, Singapore, Malaysia and Japan where we helped put a stamp of youth leadership on the environmental movement. The next year Bill arranged for me to lead a group of eighteen high school students to the Earth Summit in Rio de Janeiro followed by a six-week trip throughout Brazil, again meeting with youth, leaders, even parliamentarians throughout the country. Earth Corps was definitely on the map.

Back in Seattle I happened to see a small article in *Time Magazine* about a new program being launched in Washington, DC, called Earth Corps, led by a man named Jack Wheeler. I called Jack to encourage him to choose a new name for his program, as Earth Corps was already taken. After a struggle with Jack's big ego during three insufferably long days with him in DC (he'd gone to West Point, served several presidents and been chairman of the Vietnam Memorial committee) I returned to Seattle with the Earth Corps name intact. I never heard from Jack again.

After Rio I left the YMCA for the University of Washington to help teachers learn how to teach Native American students. Fortunately, I was able to enter graduate school in anthropology to learn something about the people with whom I was working. My dissertation in 1998 emphasized collaborative work in science and math across cultural boundaries.

Many years later, one Sunday morning in early 2011, Doug looked up from the paper and asked, "What was the name of that guy you ran into in Washington, DC, when you were working with the YMCA Earth Corps?" "Jack Wheeler," I answered. Doug drew my attention to an article about the strange discovery of a body in a dumpster in Delaware. Apparent homicide. Jack Wheeler had met an untimely end, which I think remains a mystery to this day.

Jack Wheeler in a dumpster certainly merited a phone call to my former boss, Jennifer Parker, followed by a luncheon and a tour of the Seattle YMCA, culminating with a visit with the CEO, Bob Gilbertson, who knew about PFP and was eager to support it, not only in Seattle but throughout the United States. (Bill Sieverling had succumbed to cancer in the interim.) Had it not been for Jack's untimely end, the YMCA and PFP might not have made the connection.

Having learned many lessons from my first foray into the world of partnerships, my lawyer husband Doug worked with Jay Alberts and the YMCA to draft a licensing agreement that allowed the YMCA to use the PFP trademark if it followed the PFP cycling protocols. The stage was set for a major national proliferation of Pedaling For Parkinson's programs at the YMCA and other host organizations. By working carefully with existing organizations, PFP is sustainable.

Chapter 18. Brother Doug and ALS

My relationship with my middle brother, Doug, could be described as rocky at best. At worst (in a dispute about a jointly owned family property) he pointed his finger in my face and growled with a steely voice, "I hate you!"

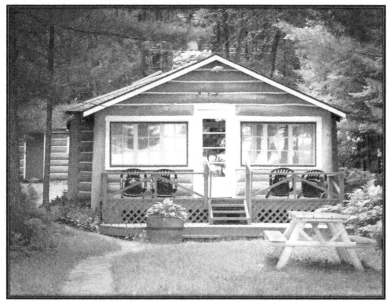

Beloved Family cottage (Photo by Doug Little)

But when he learned of my Parkinson's diagnosis, that all began to change. After my diagnosis he sent thoughtful e-mails, sharing information about the disease and strategies I might find helpful for dealing with it. He clearly cared. A side of my brother emerged that I hadn't seen since I was a child.

An even more significant change occurred when he began experiencing symptoms of Lou Gehrig's disease (ALS), his body mimicking our dad's early symptoms from nearly forty years ago. Shortly before I left for Kilimanjaro, when it was clear Doug was compromised severely, he received the formal death sentence of ALS. Unwilling to give in without a fight, since he knew bicycling had helped me, he made it a point to go to the YMCA nearly every single day to ride a spin cycle.

I called him at least each week to talk about how he was doing and see if I could offer any assistance. I listened as he begged me to find a cure or a study he could be part of. "Just a pill, Nan, please find a pill." "I don't want to die." "I don't want to die." "Please help me, Nan." Knowing full well the futility of my efforts, confirming my suspicions, I learned repeatedly as I searched that a short life expectancy disqualified him from trials. With his aggressive bulbar ALS, he would suffocate sooner rather than later.

At one point I became aware of a leading ALS researcher, Dr. Eva Feldman, at the University of Michigan. Although Dr. Feldman's lab assured me yet again that my brother Doug was not eligible for any trial study, it was important to Doug and to me to get an appointment for him there. No one returned my calls. Frustrated and demoralized by running into virtual walls, I decided to play my trump card, my doctorate. No need to disclose I was an anthropologist; I was Dr. Little. I called Dr. Feldman's office, and upon hearing Dr. Little was calling, they connected me with Dr. Ann Little. Dr. Nan Little (anthropologist) conversed about ALS with Dr. Ann Little (neurologist). It took less than five minutes before the other Dr. Little paused and asked, "So what kind of doctor are you anyway?" I had been honest about having a doctorate; we both had a good laugh. She said if she ever has a question about anthropology, I will be the first source she calls. Two days later Doug spent several hours with Dr. Little, who confirmed there was really nothing to be done. Despite knowing ahead of time the futility of my efforts, both he and I were satisfied we had covered all the bases.

At Northwestern University we connected with a lab working on genetic studies of familial neurodegenerative diseases. Because we had two people with ALS in our family and one with Parkinson's, they asked my brothers and me to donate blood samples for their databank, which we did after the memorial service for Mom.

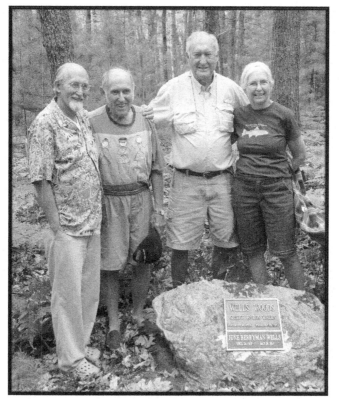

Siblings: Bob, Doug, Tom and Nan
(Photo by Doug Little)

My husband and I met Doug at a hospital to facilitate the donation. It was hard to leave, very hard, knowing when we said goodbye we would probably never see each other again. And that was the case. We walked to the parking lot together, held each other and cried, choked quietly "I love you" over and over and finally, with tears streaming off our cheeks, walked to our respective cars and headed to home and to the airport, sobbing. Over the course of the last several months my brother and I had run the gamut from sentiments of hate and disrespect, jealousy, mocking each other, not really caring to know each other, to rediscovering and affirming the love of our family. I believe our parents would have been pleased.

I learned a lot about death and dying over the next several months. It seemed to me that no matter what I or anyone else thought, the only person who had anything truly important to say about the manner of his dying was brother Doug. We should respect his wishes. Although it was clear he would benefit from being with hospice or in an assisted living situation or even having a caretaker, he wanted none of the above. He was happy in his own way, enjoying the view from his apartment and trying to do the best he could for himself. He insisted on pedaling at the YMCA almost every day. Once he fell off the bike at the Y and cut himself badly, but he didn't complain and shortly returned to his pedaling lifeline. I encouraged him to keep moving and eating even though both became increasingly challenging. He dropped from nearly 200 lbs. to less than 120, prompting him to ask how much Dad weighed when he died, as though he believed when he reached Dad's number, his own number was up.

We talked about little things that were problematic, areas where I could help to some degree. Elastic and Velcro became his best friends: buttons and zippers lost stature. He appreciated the advice. Since we both had neurodegenerative diseases, barriers faded. We talked as we never had talked before, even though his voice changed rapidly, and in a matter of a few months I could barely parse out his sentences. Everything was shutting down. I treasured the calls, realizing that in triaging life experiences, petty squabbles meant nothing, especially when contrasted with a legacy of love.

Doug arranged to call one of his friends three times a day at specific times, and if he didn't call, she was to call the front desk of his apartment building and ask someone go to his apartment to see if he was alive. That way, he figured, if he'd fallen or he was injured in some way, someone would come fairly soon to help him out, and if he were dead, at least he wouldn't lie there long.

He kept his sense of humor, odd as it was. At one point he whispered to me, slowly choking out his words, one by one, "Well, Nan, I think I'm going to know pretty soon if I'm going to heaven or going to hell." I told him I didn't believe in heaven and hell, but it was important he feel he had lived the life he wanted to live, and that was good enough. He told me he took comfort in my words.

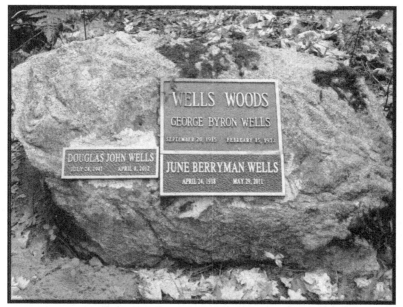

Memorial rock at Michigan cottage

By early spring it was evident his time was short. I tried to honor what he wanted, which he told me was simply to be left alone in his apartment, hopefully seated in his recliner chair watching a golf tournament while he slipped away quietly and peacefully. On Easter Sunday, Doug didn't call his friend. She called the front desk and they found him barely breathing, tilted in his recliner with the Masters Tournament on TV, exactly as he had wanted.

Doug and I had talked a great deal about donating his brain for research. He had no children, but a sample of his brain might help researchers untangle mysteries of family genetic propensity to neural degeneration. I had sent Doug a pamphlet about brain donations that the ALS researchers in Ann Arbor had sent me along with my carefully reasoned rationale for signing up for my personal donation. He answered simply. "Let's do it. Luv Doug." I wept at his response. He died Easter Sunday, April 8, 2012.

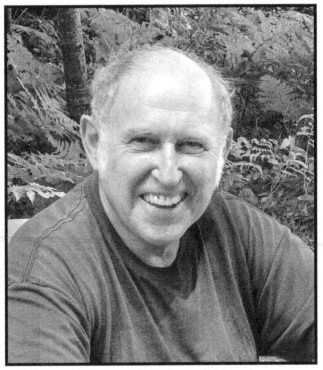

Douglas Wells, my middle brother

The only thing he seemed to care about at the end was that his life and death had meaning. He wanted his brain donated for ALS research. With the assistance of many hospital staff in Mobile and Ann Arbor, I spent much of that Easter coordinating the donation. Hopefully that research will have an impact on his nephews and nieces and grandnieces and grandnephews and everyone else in the world with that horrible disease. Months later I received a note from Dr. Eva Feldman, thanking me for the donation.

I learned a lot from my brother. I hope I'm able to apply it when my turn comes. Some holidays you won't forget. That Easter Sunday was one of them.

Chapter 19. Annapurna Base Camp Trek, May 2012

All the while I was dealing with the issues surrounding brother Doug and his ALS, I was training for a trek in Nepal. When my husband was not able to summit Mount Kilimanjaro, he wondered if it was because of his chest congestion compounded by lack of sleep or if there was some physical limitation that kept him from climbing high. When the opportunity arose to trek to Annapurna Base Camp in Nepal (13,550 feet) with an alumni group from Princeton, he asked if I wanted to go. Since Doug asked for very few things, I tried to say "yes" whenever possible.

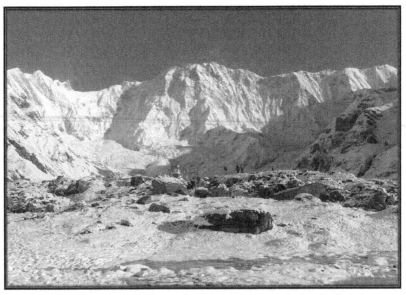

Part of the Annapurna range (Photo by Doug Little)

The program, "Rocks and Docs", was led by a son-father team: Blair Schoene, Assistant Professor of Geosciences at Princeton, and his dad, Princeton grad, Dr. Robert (Brownie) Schoene, noted high altitude medical expert. Trekking the

Himalaya with a geologist and a high altitude doctor. What could be better? We signed up.

We didn't have much time to train for the early May trip. Although we climbed steps and rode inside through the rainy winter, I didn't do the core training I had done for Kilimanjaro. Between working with PFP, taking care of our baby grandchildren and trying to find something to help my brother with his ALS, I was a mess, but I determined to try to reach Annapurna Base Camp.

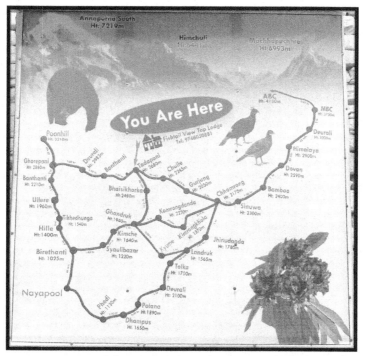

Map of the trek (Photo by Doug Little)

Despite the deaths of both my mother and my brother in a ten-month period, in many ways the Annapurna Base Camp trek was the most wonderful trip of my life. Since I was the only one in the group with a neurodegenerative disease, we didn't talk about Parkinson's incessantly, or actually much at all. I didn't realize how much I needed a break from disease conversations. (As did Doug.)

♫ ♫ ♫ ♫ ♫

On the very first day it became apparent to one of the young guides, Mohan, that I would probably need extra help. He asked the lead guide if it would be all right to stick with me. Given permission, he stayed at my elbow the entire trek, watching that I did not slip or stumble or fall too far behind.

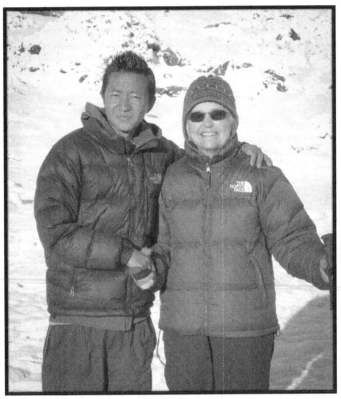

Mohan, the perfect guide (Photo by Doug Little)

On the second day, when Mohan offered to carry my pack, too proud, I told him no. Since we fell further and further behind, he finally suggested that he take some of the stuff out of my pack, including my jackets, which he tucked into the stretch cords on the back of his pack. About half an hour later, when we stopped for a break, we realized my red Gore-Tex rain jacket was missing.

Devastated, Mohan ran back down the path as fast as he could go, but it was clear to both of us the jacket would not be found. When he returned empty-handed, he was so apologetic that he was almost in tears. I reassured him that someone else needed the jacket more than I did and that other people in our group had jackets, so not to worry. I still had my lightweight jacket with me in case it turned cold.

We had lagged a bit behind the group before; we were nearly an hour behind after the jacket incident. Nervously, we looked back down the valley and saw deep black clouds rolling toward us. No gentle Seattle rain; this promised to be a deluge, a very cold deluge as the temperature dropped over 20 degrees. Along with my lightweight jacket, I carried a small umbrella for moments when I needed privacy, not much of a barrier from heavy rainfall. Both helped as the rain sheeted down, but neither did the trick.

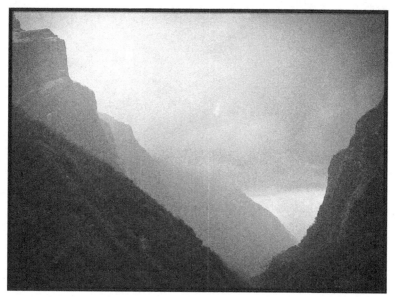

Storm moving up the valley (Photo by Doug Little)

Fortunately we came upon a small windowless stone cabin tucked alongside the trail. One of our porters had his head in the door, asking the owner for refuge. Mohan pushed past and entered the cabin to explain the situation. In a heartbeat I was sitting on a white plastic chair out of the rain, in front of a cozy fire that provided both light and heat.

The woman of indeterminate age who owned the cabin sat cross-legged on a raised platform. Next to her burned a small fire over which was balanced a pot of water. She offered us tea. The walls were lined with shelves filled with bottles and pans and very little food. Underneath one of the shelves rested a bamboo cage, with a chicken cackling inside, adding its clamor to the cacophony of noise from the rain on the roof. A small opening led to another room in which I could see piles of straw, which I presumed she used for her bed. Mohan and I occupied the two guest chairs.

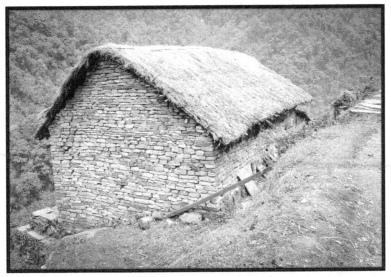

Typical hut by the path (Photo by Doug Little)

I thought the room was already full, but we were quickly joined by all ten of our porters and then by Marvin, the senior member of our trekking group. The hut, about 10 feet by 10 feet, hardly gave us room to breathe, but plenty of room to laugh. We stayed, much like the proverbial sardines in a can, for at least half an hour. Finally the rain let up enough for the porters to move on, leaving Marvin, Mohan and me with our hostess. We gave her Marvin's candy bar, and I gave her my bandana, which she proudly tied around her head, grinning from ear to ear. When the rain finally abated we left, safe and warm, the owners of a new story while someone else owned a new rain jacket and our hostess sported a red bandana.

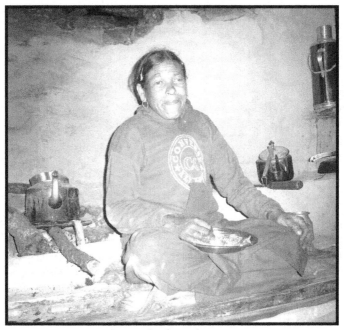

Hostess during the storm

After the storm on the first day, we learned it was in our best interest to look behind us down the valley to estimate how much time we might have before the cold rains blotted out the landscape. The days often started cool but bright, and then warmed to clear sunshine with glorious views before clouding over and lashing us with ever-colder rains that turned to hail and eventually snow as we ascended.

Mohan and I would eat lunch and be on our way as soon as possible to try to get to our teahouse stocked with hot tea, beer and Pringles while we were still dry. Each teahouse had separate rooms with two to five beds, generally two bathrooms (Western or not), and a large communal area for eating, hanging out and listening to university level presentations on geology and medicine. Our professors even brought a whiteboard to illustrate their lectures.

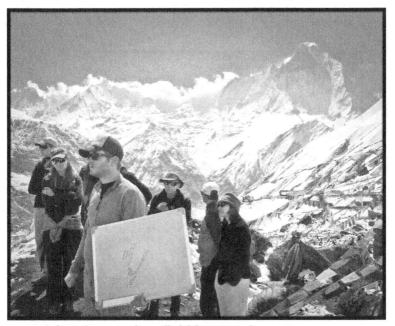

Blair Schoene gives field lecture above Annapurna
Base Camp with Machhapuchhre in background
(Photo by Doug Little)

One afternoon as I was setting up our room, I heard voices on the walkway outside. Two young women and a man, having misjudged the storm, had just arrived at our teahouse thoroughly drenched and freezing cold, on the edge of hypothermia. These French Canadians had not arranged for accommodations ahead of time and were out of luck at this particular teahouse, as our group filled all the spaces. I invited them into our room and told them to put on something warm and dry, then go to the teahouse meeting room and have some warm drinks before heading further up the mountain. They gratefully complied.

As the young man was changing his shirt, he explained in his halting English that he needed to leave the women to go

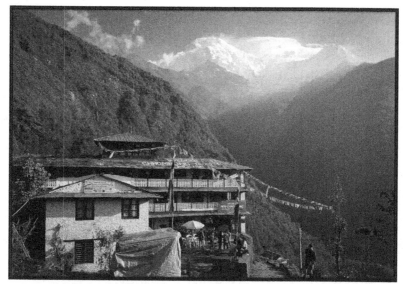

Fancy teahouse at Chomrong with view of
Annapurna South and Machhapuchhre
(Photo by Doug Little)

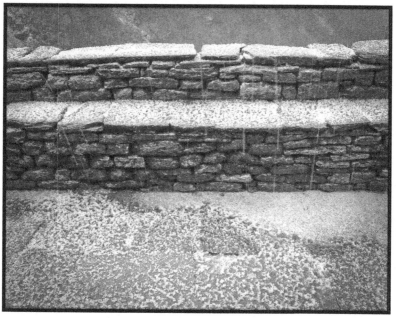

Daily afternoon hailstorm
(Photo by Doug Little)

further up to secure a place to stay and then come back and get them. It was particularly hard, I needed to understand, because he had Parkinson's disease and he didn't have the stamina he once had. We spent the next fifteen minutes talking about PFP and strategies for taking charge of his own life. How unexpected, to be able to offer comfort, strategy and hope to a fellow traveler in the mountains of Nepal in a driving rainstorm.

We ascended and descended thousands of intricately fitted stone steps.

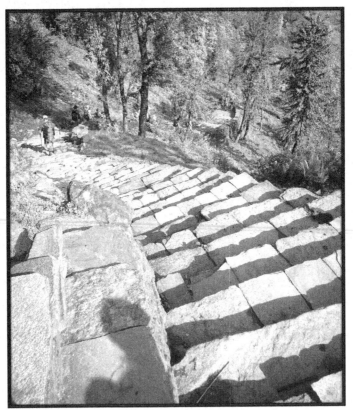

Up steps. Down steps.
Along the trail to Annapurna Base Camp
(Photo by Doug Little)

Scenery, companions (ages twenty-three to seventy, including six doctors and a medical student) and Nepalese guides made the trip. In the Annapurna Sanctuary with mountains looming, I knew I was on holy ground. I stopped several times with Mohan just to cry at the beauty and wonder of the place and the experience.

I felt enveloped by place. Once again I was not alone, even though many times Mohan and I were the only ones from our group visible on the trail.

Often I stopped in the middle of a swaying bridge over a wildly pulsating mountain river. When Mohan encouraged me not to be afraid, I explained to his amazement that I stopped on wobbly bridges on purpose to marvel at the power of nature and to absorb as much of the experience as possible.

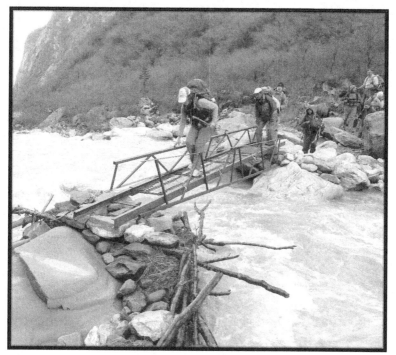

Crossing the Modi Khola
on a non-OSHA-approved bridge
(Photo by Doug Little)

❧ ❧ ❧ ❧ ❧

Although I had developed a herniated disc and several cysts on my vertebrae (reminiscent of RAGBRAI) at the beginning of the Nepal trek, the pain seldom interfered with my engagement with the place and people. I discovered that if I could lie on my back and pedal into the air at every break, the action relieved the pressure on my spine enough to enable me to hike the next segment with a low level of pain. Thinking outside of myself, outside of my concerns for Parkinson's and my future, enabled me to draw on parts of me that are courageous, tenacious and loving.

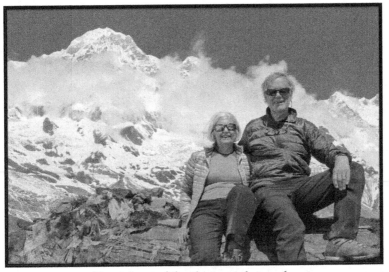

Together with place and people
Annapurna South in background

The more I focused on pain, things I could no longer do, or ramifications of having Parkinson's, the more debilitated and closed in I became. Parkinson's was a bother, but the more I did, the more I realized it was true that, for that moment at least, although I had a disease, I was not sick.

I carried two banners to the Annapurna Base Camp and made wall hangings of them when we returned. One was for Doug and commemorated both the trek and Pedaling For Parkinson's. The other was to raise funds at the American Parkinson's Disease Association auction.

The banner that sold at the auction represented the Hope that people in the PD community have for a cure and the hope we have for the strength to deal with daily challenges. It honored people with Parkinson's, our caregivers, and the professional community that helps us. It also helped us remember those who went before, including my mother and brother, who had both died so recently. Every stitch was sewn with love.

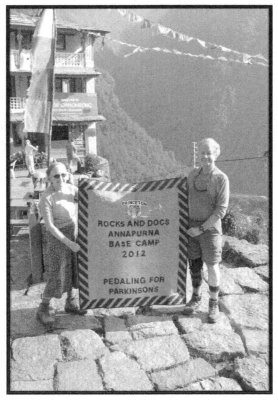

Banner celebrating the trek and
Pedaling For Parkinson's

Although some members of the Annapurna group suffered from low-level headaches, neither Doug nor I experienced any difficulties, confirming his hypothesis that the problems he endured on Kilimanjaro resulted from the congestion of his cold rather than acute mountain sickness. This left us confident that we could participate in other treks if the opportunity arose. Opportunities abound.

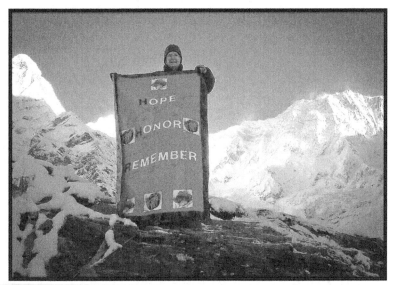

PD banner: Hope, Honor, Remember
(Photo by Doug Little)

Chapter 20. RAGBRAI 2012, July 21-27

Despite my herniated disc and cysts on my vertebrae, shortly after we returned from Nepal in early May we travelled to the east coast, then headed to Colorado for a Kilimanjaro reunion, followed by the RAGBRAI ride across Iowa in July. Thanks to the heroic efforts of my physical therapist and a lot of hard work on my part, I was back on my bike within two weeks of our return from Nepal, nearly pain free, but under clear restrictions as to how much I was to cycle before Iowa. Consequently, I started RAGBRAI with almost no cycling preparation, not a good idea with a brutal heat wave engulfing the entire center section of the United States.

We encountered the oppressive, enervating heat in Hull, Iowa, the gathering spot for the PFP group of RAGBRAI riders. It was so hot I even used thinning shears to rid our long-haired miniature dachshunds of some of their dense hair. They still suffered all week, maybe more than the rest of us, but at least they were well loved by all the children in our group. Again, it was good to see old friends and meet new. Of the five of us with PD, all but me were young-onset; all courageous strong people, eager to share the message that PD does not necessarily need to be the sentence to a life of misery it once was. John and I were old hands, this being our third RAGBRAI. Karen and Cidney had both ridden in 2011, and this was Bob's first effort at RAGBRAI.

Day 1: Hot

"We rode 63.47 miles today. The temperature was 96 degrees in late afternoon. I drank seven 20-ounce bottles of water and went to the bathroom once. What more needs to be said?"

Day 2: Chaos and Survival

"We rode 64.23 miles. The temperature was 105 degrees late in the evening, but it had been up to 115 degrees during the day when measured above the road, and 126 degrees at road level.

"This was the most chaotic day I can recall in any RAGBRAI. Terrible heat. Radio, television and newspaper reporters all suggested that for our safety we should not ride in the intense heat. Most rode anyway. This was not fun; it was endurance heaped upon endurance. I wished for breezes, but each time I felt a little wind, it just blew hotter air against my body. I felt as if I was opening an oven door but I couldn't close it, my feet rooted to the spot so the heat couldn't be avoided.

"My strategy, like everyone else's, was to start as early in the morning as possible, take few breaks and drink as much as I could force into my body. This was not laughable. It was serious business. Like the cold on Kilimanjaro, this heat was beyond anything I had ever encountered; I hoped to never encounter it again. I ran into my ever-patient and strong teammate, Rene, and we helped each other along. It was great to be riding with a friend who had such encouraging words. Each town was packed as people tried to eat and drink as much as possible while resting in the dry heat. I expect they were all rather dreading getting back on their bikes. I was.

"Around lunchtime Rene and I ran into one of Jay's staffers looking for her twelve-year-old son, Sam, who was lost somewhere in the middle of this tightly packed mass of people. She was frantic. Rene and I assured her we would keep our eyes out for him. When we found him, we invited him to join us, and then called his mom to assure her he was safe. Although it felt good to eat and rest in the shade, the heat was intensifying and it would get hotter yet. We three needed to go.

"For whatever reasons, apparently not related to Parkinson's, I did not feel at all well when we left town. I found it hard to keep my natural pace when I was watching out for Sam; Rene was watching out for both of us; and Sam was watching out for me too. We all had reason to be concerned. I could tell I was slowing them down, not a good thing on this particular day. Needing to set my own pace, I told them to ride off together and I would be fine. Sam and Rene had already kept me going for several hours. As they left, Sam looked back sorrowfully until I was out of sight. Later his mom told me he suffered for months, concerned he had abandoned me in my time of need.

"With just three miles to go, I realized something was very wrong. As I slowly pumped up the last hill, my heart rate jumped from 135 to 147 in one rotation of the pedals. This was not Potter's Hill revisited but something far more serious. Head spinning, I unclipped my pedals, dismounted awkwardly, put my head on my handlebars, and tried to push the bike up the hill. I recall many people asking if I was okay and my numbly telling them yes. Fortunately our two doctor riders happened along and joined me. We stumbled 25 yards to an ice water stand. When I asked if I could sit, there must have been something in my voice, because in no time I was plopped in a bucket chair, draped with ice-water towels, and packed in ice: front and back, neck, armpits, crotch. Oddly enough, I never felt cold the hour I curled up buried in ice cubes. Close to a heat stroke, the doctors assured me if I had ridden the last three miles I would have spent the night in a hospital or a morgue. Scary.

"During that whole sequence of icy events I was more concerned about my IPod and dumb phone soaking in ice water in my back pocket than about PD. (At the end of the day both still worked!)"

Day 3: More Heat, Time to Sag

"I drove our van today. It was the first time I had ever sagged on RAGBRAI, giving me a different way of getting to know the trip and learning what makes it work behind the scenes. It's an operation powered by utterly calm, capable people: Iowans.

"The heat kept rising, with reports of the heat index at 115 degrees and road surface temperatures at 127 degrees. Many in our group kept riding the whole time, including Doug. I had noted the day before that the tar used to fill cracks in the road was melting and should be avoided. Although we heard lots of ambulances, it appeared no one was seriously injured."

Day 4: Another Close Call

"Much of the same, only more people sagged at least part of the day. Seven children stuffed into the back of the van; one adult sat next to me in the front. Of the four seatbelts, only the front two were buckled. Suddenly I heard a flop, flop, flop sound. Worrisome. The other adult insisted it was just my tires hitting the rumbles, but I knew in my gut something was wrong with our van. As we were on the freeway at the time, I stupidly kept driving, hoping we would exit shortly. Last in the line of four vehicles, I did not know where we were going, nor did I have a phone number for any of the other drivers. The tremor in my hand went wild, making almost as much noise as the flopping outside. Fortunately the tire tread held to the exit and then to the nearby midday meeting point, where I saw tread separated from the tire, just a hairs' breadth from causing a blowout. It could have been awful, but since nothing bad actually happened it became another PFP RAGBRAI story. When Doug happened to stop at the midway point, he took over the tire issue.

"Once I realized the potential disaster that had been averted, I fell apart thinking about what might have happened if the tire had blown with all those unbelted children inside. After a few private tears I was back to my game face and able to drive. We bought two new rear tires and much peace of mind.

"Storms finally came through during the night, dropping the temperature about 20 degrees—still hot, but more within reason. Our group slept in an air-conditioned American Legion Hall basement while Doug and I and the dogs watched the clouds and felt the wind from inside the van. Exhausted from the recent traumas, I actually fell asleep during the storm!"

Day 5: Get Back in the Saddle

"I felt well enough to ride, but deciding 80 miles might be a bit much, I drove to the midpoint and rode from there. While worried about getting back on the bike, I realized if I didn't do it then I might not muster the courage to ever do it. Since my quality of life depends on my being able to ride to health, I climbed aboard and did just fine. I forgot to write down all the stats, but as I recall, I rode about 45 miles without incident."

Day 6: Accident

"Today was the shortest day on the ride, just 48 miles. Though still quite warm, the searing heat was a thing of the past. I enjoyed many hills, light winds, and the glorious feeling of doing something again to make myself more well.

"Sadly and painfully, just as they were entering the final town, Cidney's husband veered into her wheel. She fell hard, badly breaking her wrist and scraping multiple body parts. Despite a broken wrist and PD, Cid kept an unbelievably upbeat attitude. We often say we can't control what happens to us, but we can control our attitude. Cid exemplified the attitude I wish I had all the time. What a trooper! After spending hours in the hospital, she endured a long, painful night tucked in a reclining chair in the gracious and helpful local nursing home that hosted us the final night. With no showers available, residents opened their rooms to let us clean up and staff let us use their laundry facilities. They also fed us. I expect we were the source of conversation for the next several months. Nursing home residents hold a warm place in my heart. I hope I remember these gracious Iowans when it's my turn."

Day 7: Deflated

"The final ride is generally a short day as everyone is eager to get started toward home. After the week of heat and close calls, hardly anyone wanted to take the time to ride all 70 miles. Quite a few of our group left last night. Since Doug and I were taking Cid and her husband to the airport, we rode only half the route. We didn't need to prove anything."

♪ ♪ ♪ ♪ ♪

Not enough can be said about the generous hospitality we received everywhere we stayed. People came to hear us speak. Staff fed us and helped with our laundry. People eagerly listened to our stories and cheered us on. The PFP staff was always generous and calm no matter what the crisis. They have my applause and gratitude.

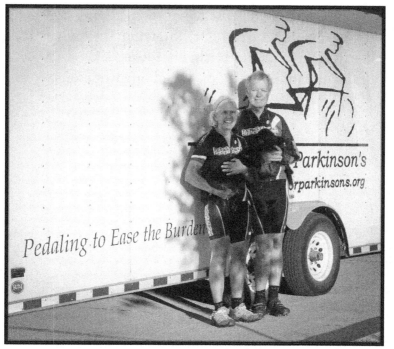

RAGBRAI 2012, Final day

This was a hard RAGBRAI for me: hard because of the heat, hard because I wasn't prepared and hard because I hadn't recovered from the Annapurna trip enough to have my symptoms under control. It proved to me without a doubt I must keep a regular riding regimen if I'm to be on top of this disease. There is no faking it for me. Ride the bike or ride the wheelchair. Take my pick.

As the oldest woman in the group and the oldest with PD, in my low moments I felt somewhat isolated, more like a mom or grandma than a participant among buddies. On the other hand, I talked with ever so many people who were eager to know about PFP and I fielded many requests for information before we even finished the ride.

I didn't know if I would do it again. Surely three trips across Iowa, standing on top of Mount Kilimanjaro and trekking thousands of steps to Annapurna Base Camp should be sufficient evidence of the efficacy of the pedaling program. PFP worked for me, for sure. But, knowing me, when the next opportunity arose, I would be there. I was.

In the meantime, I encountered other demons.

Chapter 21. REM Sleep Behavior Disorder

Even before I was diagnosed with Parkinson's, violent dreams had interrupted our nights, with me frequently threatening to attack Doug, or just screaming and thrashing in my sleep. Most nights I fended off imaginary attackers who were all too real to me. My "role" was to defend and prevent harm from coming near us. All too often my husband awoke to screeches and my fist swinging violently as I hit and kicked these phantoms. Fortunately, Doug avoided the brunt of this violence, more than once grabbing my wrist just before I could smash my fist in his face. In my dreams he often represented a threatening stranger. Once, in our camper van, the threat was so dangerously imminent I punched my fist as hard as I could into the side of the van. It's a wonder I didn't break either my hand or the van. I would remember these dreams vividly the next morning, and I often wrote them down. It is still scary to read about the large men who appeared in our bedroom before melting away and showing up elsewhere.

Violent dreams continued, unabated, after I was diagnosed with Parkinson's. They became so out of hand, bizarre and dangerous that Dr. Roberts recommended I meet with a sleep disorder specialist who put me through a remarkable test to determine if I had REM sleep behavior disorder, another unfortunate selection on the menu of undesirable options for PwPs. Like loss of the sense of smell, acting out REM dreams may be an early indicator of Parkinson's.

Late one night I carried my overnight bag through dimly lighted hospital halls heading to the Sleep Disorder Center as though I were on my way to a slumber party. The tech took her time explaining what was going to happen before attaching a multitude of electrodes to my scalp, my body, around my chest and legs, everywhere. I looked and felt like a Halloween alien octopus. I wondered how I would be able to sleep with all the hardware attached to my body. She assured me that a sleeping pill would solve that problem and she would spend the whole night watching my brain waves bounce around on the computer, like a seismograph responding to earthquakes. Not a slumber party.

I swallowed the pill, curled up under the covers and dimly noted the lights going out. When I awoke about 4:00 a.m., she explained I had finished my REM sleep; they had their data. She chuckled and said when I entered REM sleep I started to bicycle like mad, legs flailing in circles like I was pedaling. For some unknown reason I did not exhibit the violent side of my REM sleep behavior disorder. Nonetheless, my bicycling activity confirmed the diagnosis.

The sleep doctor gave me the bad news that PwPs who have this disorder have an increased likelihood of developing Lewy body dementia. I had heard that the prospect of developing this dementia ranged from as much as 95% to more conservative estimates of 50%. Neither was a pretty prospect. Usually REM sleep behavior disorder manifested itself many years before the actual onset of other Parkinson's symptoms. Mine manifested itself just a few years before diagnosis. I was a bit of an anomaly. Nothing new there.

The doctor skimmed over the part about dementia to focus on positive aspects of my diagnosis. There were few, or at least few I could see. He could give me a pill to help with my insomnia and the crazy night behaviors. If the drug worked well, my husband, the van and I would all be safe. That sounded good, so I filled the prescription for clonazepam and entered yet another phase of my life as a drug addict. If I stopped taking clonazepam, I would be hurting for sure. Every night I dutifully took my pill; I nearly always got a good night's sleep, everyone was safe and I didn't lie awake worrying about going crazy.

About every six months my sleep doctor invited me in for a little talk to see how I was doing. Most of the time we talked about Montana and fly-fishing. He asked how I was sleeping, and I explained that when there was an especially stressful time I increased my dose to one and a half pills, and then reduced it to one and a quarter pills, and then went back to one pill when it felt right. These pills were only 0.5 mg, so it didn't seem to me I was increasing or reducing by much. I realized I was getting better and better at self-diagnosis. He approved.

Because REM sleep events are exacerbated by any external stress, it was no surprise that one of my worst experiences was the night after my mother's memorial service. My niece had arranged for us to stay at the lovely home of her friends in Ann Arbor. Although the service had gone well and I was happy with how it all turned out, I knew I was highly stressed. Sure enough, in the middle of the night a woman came into our bedroom to attack us. As she came toward the bed I yelled at her to get out of our room. Apparently my screaming was just garbled noise, but then I kicked—I kicked at her as hard as I could, but I didn't hit her. So I kicked again, with all my might, and kicked myself right out of the bed, slamming my hip into the side rail as I fell into the disheveled pile of quilts. The pain was unbelievable. I thought for sure I had cracked a bone, and to this day I don't know if I did or not. The bruise lasted well over a month covering a hard knot the size of a golf ball that ached for weeks.

When my brother, Doug, died ten months after Mom, we had his memorial service in Michigan in August 2012, almost exactly a year after hers. I took an extra half pill to ensure I would sleep through each night. At home I titrated myself back to one and a quarter pills and then down to one without any difficulty at all.

♫ ♫ ♫ ♫ ♫

Having control of my own life is tremendously important, even more important now than ever before. I expect it's related to my initial reaction on hearing I had Parkinson's disease: the overwhelming feeling of being on an ice sheet without an ice ax to arrest my slippery slide. In the course of one sentence I had gone from being a member of the human race to being a member of a medical subset. From that moment on, too many decisions would be made *for* me rather than *with* me. It didn't feel right. It certainly didn't feel good.

I don't believe I am fated to have one life or another. I don't believe a God decided I would have Parkinson's, or that my dad and my brother would have ALS and my other two brothers would be just fine. I don't believe anyone ever did anything to deserve Parkinson's or ALS or any other nasty in the alphabet soup of diseases. I don't believe we were chosen because we had the strength to deal with this crisis. Things happen over which none of us have control, but we can and do control how we deal with them. That's what I mean about having control over my own life.

Chapter 22. Sips of Lemonade

Having a disability, being a member of a medical subset, puts one in a special relationship with others in the same boat. Moments like the following reaffirm our connections.

🐾 🐾 🐾 🐾 🐾

We met up with fishing friends of Doug's in Bozeman, Montana. She had cancer. I note how people who have a disease that makes their clock tick a little faster manage to cut right to the chase. Even though we had never met before, in no time we felt like old friends. There is a bond I never realized existed until I became one of those who feel every minute of every day is somehow hallowed. We don't have time to build friendships over years; we either click or we move on. We clicked. In 2013, sadly, she moved on.

🐾 🐾 🐾 🐾 🐾

I met a one-armed fisherman in the river. I watched for a while before offering to help take the fly out of his fish. I asked how he does it with one arm, and he explained he uses hemostats most of the time. I explained, "I have Parkinson's and sometimes it's really tough for me to get the fly out too." He laughed and said, "Especially when it's cold. Eh?" Quite so. Shared disabilities—a new club.

🐾 🐾 🐾 🐾 🐾

We were fishing a lesser-known spot on the South Fork of the Madison River near West Yellowstone. I watched another angler drive in and arrange an elaborate setup for putting on his gear. It looked familiar, since I employ similar techniques to climb into my gear. I went over and commented that we have something in common. He looked at me quizzically and asked what that might be. I pointed out that both of us have tremor-dominant Parkinson's. He got a little huffy and told me he didn't have Parkinson's. "Oh, sorry," I said and continued on to the river to fish.

The next year I saw him at a charity fundraiser for the West Yellowstone Historical Center. I went over to chat, and he commented on my tremor and said that he, too, had Parkinson's. "It was the darndest thing," he said. "I didn't know I had Parkinson's until last year I was out on the South Fork and some lady came up and told me I had it. She diagnosed me right there on the river. I went to my doctor and she was right!"

I confessed. He thanked me.

♪ ♪ ♪ ♪ ♪

"Hi, my name is Glenn Erickson [bike racer and custom frame builder] and I have Parkinson's. I put on a little fundraising bike ride each year and I'd like the money to help people with Parkinson's here in the northwest. I hear you have a cycling program for PwPs. Maybe we could work together." The first Glenn Erickson Pedaling For Parkinson's ride in 2013 raised over $10,000 to train YMCA staff to run PFP programs. Another $10,000 at the 2014 ride. I never know who will be on the other end of the line.

Chapter 23. Medicine Mess

By the fall of 2012 I had already thrown the dart at just about all available dopamine agonists and Parkinson's medications except for Sinemet, the combination of Carbidopa and Levodopa, which has for decades been the gold standard for most patients. I was so afraid of developing dyskinesias, those unpredictable jerky movements, that I avoided the medicine. After we returned from our customary fishing trip to Yellowstone and Silver Creek, Idaho in the fall of 2012, unbeknownst to me a generic form of Requip XL had been developed and distributed to pharmacies to pass on to patients. When the mail order pharmacy sent me the generic instead of the brand-name drug, I didn't pay much attention to the change; I had a different-colored pill and the bottle said Ropinerole instead of Requip XL.

With my new pills I almost immediately felt nauseous for a couple of hours each day. Then the couple extended to three, four, and up to six hours. Every day I would wake up knowing that sometime between ten o'clock and noon I would start feeling nausea that would last until almost dinnertime. My high energy level plummeted. Every single day I wanted to nap for hours. But I had things to do, grandchildren to enjoy, a life to lead, and I did not want to sleep away half of my life. I was still riding my bicycle diligently: at least an hour a day in the basement during the bad weather, and outside when the weather was good. It seemed like the only thing that kept me going was my commitment to ride my bike.

As the days went by I became more and more sick. Parkinson's was just the luck of the draw, but feeling nauseous every day seemed like something I ought to be able to avoid, especially since I had not felt ill while using the normal Requip XL. I was furious the drug had been swapped for something cheaper.   When I spoke to several people about their experiences with generic drugs, they said that for the most part they noticed very little difference, but in some cases, like mine, they had extremely negative reactions.

After suffering for a week I contacted my neurologist to show him my wildly flapping hand and explain the daily nausea. He immediately wrote a prescription for the regular Requip XL, hoping that by changing back to the familiar drug my new symptoms would disappear. That didn't happen. I tried and tried to be my normal self, but I had a totally flat affect and the nausea remained. Recognizing that the non-generic Requip XL was not going to solve my problem, we returned to the Neupro patch, which worked quite well except for the inevitable side effects and the exorbitant cost. Stomach problems were replaced by an increasing tremor in my right arm that made my arm ache, my fingers ache and the ring finger on my right hand lock up and freeze completely. Nonetheless, these problems were preferable to being on the verge of throwing up six hours a day. After three months on the Neupro patch I tried to return to Requip XL but after a month I gave up and returned to Neupro for another year.

Chapter 24. More Effective Medicine

Rosie, at age 2:

"Grandma, if you sit on your dancing hand, will it stop dancing?"

"I can help you, Grandma. I'll put a pink smiley bear tattoo on your dancing hand and you can make it stop when you want."

"Grandma, you need someone to keep you company when you take your naps. You can keep my Humpty Dumpty pillow. If you put your dancing hand under Humpty Dumpty, you can sleep better."

Rosie, at age 4:

Grandma: "Rosie, when I squeeze your hand, it means 'I love you'." Pause. Rosie: "Grandma, can I hold your dancing hand?"

A dancing hand is much more manageable than Parkinson's disease—and love is just as effective as medication.

Chapter 25. Research

Amid the many baffling twists and turns of this disease, it is clear to me that we are not going to emerge from the Parkinson's maze until the causes—not just cause, but causes—are identified. Drug developers create medicines, searching to ameliorate the condition or conditions that PwPs face. The real truth is that without biomarkers to measure the extent of change, pharmaceutical companies are shooting in the dark nearly as much as doctors and patients.

I often think of the people who spent their lives in iron lungs because those devices enabled them to breathe despite the ravages of polio. But when the cause of polio was identified and the Salk vaccine was formulated, the business of making iron lungs was over. I look at our Parkinson's medications and surgeries as modern-day iron lungs. Taking the drugs is better than suffocating or experiencing the living hell that generations before us endured. They keep us going, but drugs and brain surgeries don't and won't solve the problem.

On the "causes" front, the scientific community is looking for biological indicators that will tell if a person either has Parkinson's or has a propensity to develop the disease. People with MS have annual MRIs to determine the state of their disease. Currently, although some promising technologies are in the works, no biomarker in blood, genetic records, brain scans, or anything else allows physicians to conclusively diagnose Parkinson's or measure its progression. At research laboratories all over the world scientists are trying to understand what happens in people with Parkinson's, to both allow them to measure the efficacy of pharmaceutical and non-pharmaceutical interventions, such as exercise or surgery, or to create the Parkinson's equivalent of the Salk vaccine. The ability to know in a timely way if an intervention actually works, without waiting for autopsy, obviously will speed up the treatment phases of research.

Hope colors the horizon in the form of the Michael J. Fox Foundation's Parkinson's Progression Markers Initiative (PPMI). Hundreds of people with Parkinson's and hundreds of controls who do not have Parkinson's (including Doug) signed up to have their cerebral spinal fluid analyzed over a multiyear time frame. An important aspect of any initiative funded by the Fox Foundation is that all the data is open source so researchers from all over the world can use it to create and carry out experiments. If someone had to get Parkinson's, I thank God it was Michael J. Fox, because he is using his vision and resources to make a difference. Currently, more PPMI-type initiatives are being funded at the federal level, raising expectations that causes, and hopefully cures and new therapies will be identified.

Clinical trials, conducted in phases, are designed to determine the safety and effectiveness of a new drug or procedure in people. Each phase, with some overlap, has a primary objective with an ultimate goal of approving the drug for general use. Simply put:

Phase I	Is the treatment safe?
Phase II	Does the treatment work?
Phase III	Does the new treatment work better than the standard treatment?
Phase IV	Is the treatment safe over time?

The most difficult aspect of drug trials is convincing people to enroll. Patients are asked to take drugs that may or may not be helpful and that may, in certain circumstances, actually be harmful, or possibly the "drug" or even brain surgery may actually be a placebo. Research shows that approximately thirty percent (30%) of responses to drug interventions are due to the placebo effect. This means that if people expect the intervention to work, thirty percent of the time it will work, at least for a while. People who are willing to participate in clinical trials, both people with PD and those without the disease, can go to the Fox Trial Finder (https://foxtrialfinder.michaeljfox.org/) for easy access to information about what trials are enrolling participants and what criteria candidates need to meet.

When I started down this Parkinson's pathway, I decided I would participate in research studies that didn't involve drugs. It was easy to get on the bike, but not so easy to swallow a pill when I realized the potential magnitude of side effects. Several years later I concluded that some of us have to be lab rats. With our children grown and having already lived a wonderful life, I decided I should step forward, at least with a small step. As I became more involved in my role as lab rat, two experiences stood out: I became connected with some of the most cutting edge researchers in the field and I learned up close and personal what it meant to participate in a drug trial.

The drug trial began in February 2013. Research scientists hypothesized that a drug that was already being used to treat people with Alzheimer's would also have a positive effect on people with Parkinson's. Having passed the safety test, in this phase they checked for efficacy, measured by MRIs and lengthy cognitive exams. I was amazed. By the time I was titrated up to the full dosage, tests showed my memory had improved substantially and my confidence in social situations was light-years from what it had been. Subsequent testing through the cognitive exams showed I had improved there as well. Another friend of mine improved also. The examiners as well as People with Parkinson's were elated. When the trial was over, we were encouraged to stay on the medication. It did not take much encouragement.

However, shortly after that, everything changed. I lost complete confidence in my capacity to make decisions, even to select the clothes I would wear each day. My tremor increased dramatically. My shoulder became so painful I could hardly move.

I stopped taking the drug, and within a week my son told me I went from acting and thinking like an eighty-seven-year-old to acting and thinking like the sixty-seven-year-old that I actually was. I must admit that even though I'm not eager to participate in more drug trials, someone has to do it. I learned that just because a drug works for one neurologic disorder does not mean it necessarily will work for others, or more specifically, for me. Several of my friends are the first in the world to undergo experimental brain surgery. I'm not yet that brave.

The National Institutes of Health (NIH) in Washington, DC, is a center for academic research and medicine. When an opportunity came to join the Parkinson's Research Study Group at NIH, I volunteered. After much vetting they invited me to come to Washington DC for intake tests to see if I qualified. After being tested with various MRIs, including a powerful 7 Tesla MRI, and undergoing many cognitive exams, I was accepted as part of the pool they can draw on whenever they need research subjects. Research studies I have participated in, through NIH and other institutions, are listed in Appendix B. Because of my REM Sleep Behavior Disorder I'm frequently channeled into cognitive decline studies. Although I would rather not be on that side of the fence, I tell myself that if 95% of the people with this disorder develop dementia, some have to be in the 5% and one of those might as well be me. So I do my crosswords and Sudoku in efforts to keep my cognition intact. I try not to think about the 95% when I can't find my keys.

Participating in research is proactive; I know I'm *doing* something. Whereas cycling keeps the dragons at bay, I expect that research will eventually identify causes and cures for the disease. After spending so many hours as a lab rat, if an intervention is discovered, I hope I've earned a spot near the front of the line.

Chapter 26. Frozen Shoulder

Just because a person has Parkinson's doesn't mean she gets a "Get Out of Jail Free" card for other maladies. I had never heard of Frozen Shoulder until it became my close companion for nearly two years. Perhaps it started with the herniated disk in Nepal or too much airplane travel without enough stretching, or maybe I stressed it by climbing steep hills on my bike, or carrying packs up mountains, or lifting or gardening or typing or sewing without taking enough breaks. Who knows? The reality was that by August 2012 my orthopedic surgeon nephew easily diagnosed the problem, assured me surgery would not be a good option and encouraged me to wait it out for the next couple of years. Pain assaulted me at unexpected moments. I would put my keys in my pocket, but when I tried to extract them, intense pain prevented me from pulling my hand out, forcing me to use my left hand to move my right. I couldn't brush my teeth, stir-fry our dinner, comb my hair, cut my food or do virtually anything with my right hand. I couldn't imagine living the rest of my life like that, but I adapted as people do.

It got worse. By mid-March 2013 I was unable to write or type and by the end of the month I could no longer negotiate turns on the open road on my bike. Four cortisone shots didn't help; extensive physical therapy slowly made a difference over many months. But in early June, unable to negotiate an easy turn on to a bike trail bridge approach, I wiped out another cyclist, knocking us both down a grassy slope, breaking my wedding ring finger. Because I posed a danger on trails and roads, I stopped riding outside. (My beautiful ring had to be sawed off.)

None-the-less, on our climb to Machu Picchu in August I muddled along asking others to cut my food and provide assistance as needed even though I was able to carry my pack the entire way. The pain continued unabated through the winter of 2014, so debilitating I had to stop skiing because I couldn't even hold a ski pole in my right hand and finally couldn't use my right side at all. It appeared the time had come when I really would have to stop skiing for the rest of my life. As I recalled my fears after being diagnosed in 2008, I realized that most of them had been groundless as long as I just powered through with whatever resources were at my disposal. My bucket list had expanded as Doug and I went places and accomplished challenges we never dreamed we would face. So I could no longer ski. I still walked on the right side of the sod.

Chapter 27. Inca Trail to Machu Picchu, August 2013

After we had such a wonderful time in Nepal with the Princeton alumni group, Doug wondered if I might be up for another climb the following year. Since one of the doctors from the Nepal trip attended Yale, he was our ticket into Yale Alumni Adventures. One hundred and one years earlier, Yale faculty member Hiram Bingham had "discovered" Machu Picchu in Peru, or, more accurately, he had identified it as a significant historic archaeological site from the Inca civilization. The 2013 Yale alumni trek included hiking the Inca Trail for four days with the highest elevation, 13,800 feet, at Dead Woman's Pass, then descending to Machu Picchu on the final day. Three friends from the Annapurna trek joined the group: two doctors and a medical student.

Following our usual pattern, we flew into Lima a day early and into Cusco an additional day early to acclimate to culture and elevation change. The extra days enabled me to adjust the timing of my medication and to notice if I needed to address any unusual concerns. Not having experienced acute mountain sickness on either Kilimanjaro or the Annapurna Base Camp trek, I was surprised at how quickly I developed a headache in Cusco. At the other locations we had had a gradual increase in elevation; in Peru we went abruptly from sea level in Lima to 11,200 feet in Cusco. Eager to explore the town, we immediately set out to hike as high as we could to get an overview of the city. Mistake. The view was good; the headache was not. I finally had some limited appreciation for what others had gone through on Kilimanjaro, and to a lesser extent in Nepal.

Alerted that there was a person with Parkinson's in the group, the organizers made special arrangements to have an additional guide. Pepe had never been a guide before and had limited knowledge of English, history, flora and fauna or anything specifically related to the Incan sites. Although I spoke some Spanish, it wasn't enough to bridge our communication challenges. Unlike my Nepalese guide who had stayed glued to my elbow, Pepe often walked 30 feet ahead of me, which meant I trekked solo much of the time. Because Pepe and I left 45 minutes ahead of the main group, many times we arrived at the next stop long before the others who had stopped for mini-lectures along the way—cultural bonuses I truly missed.

Being alone with my guide had its definite advantages however. I could stop to poke around archaeological sites to my heart's content.

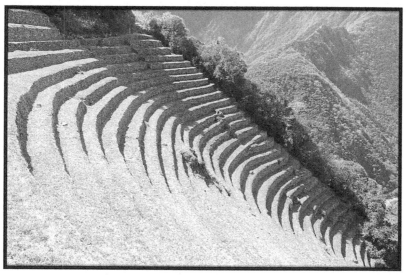

Winay Wayna site on the Inca Trail
(Photo by Doug Little)

Because we were quiet, we were able to sneak up on two exquisite giant hummingbirds (*Patagona gigas*), the largest hummingbirds in the world. Once Pepe understood I liked birds, he went out of his way to listen and to point them out, even if he did not know their names. I doubt I would have remembered them anyway. We made other "discoveries" such as a geodetic marker the rest of the group did not notice. I looked for little moments to treasure. Since I seldom needed assistance walking, our arrangement worked well.

Arriving at the lunch stops far ahead of the rest of our group, I could watch the colorful machinations of the porters putting together a feast on the trail, each person with a clearly defined role. Linens graced every table, with each napkin decoratively folded. Each outfitter on the trail wore different colors to easily identify their companies. Our porters looked handsome in burgundy and cream.

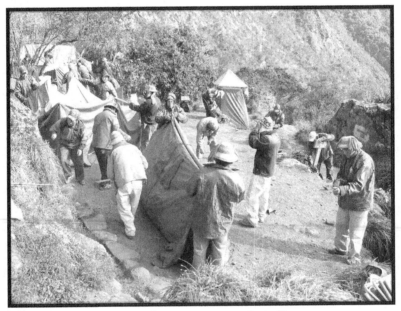

Quechua porters and staff
(Photo by Doug Little)

Since the English-speaking guides were with the rest of the group, I spent meal prep times using sign language to ask questions and make observations, thereby developing my own special bond with our crew. Other than the frozen shoulder, I felt fine as long as I took my medicine and sleeping pill.

As in Nepal, the Inca Trail was made up of thousands of steps, beautifully built into the sides of the mountains. With no guardrails and very steep drop-offs this was not a trek for the fainthearted. One woman in our group who was terrified of heights faced down her inner demons, making this trip both her personal challenge and her reward.

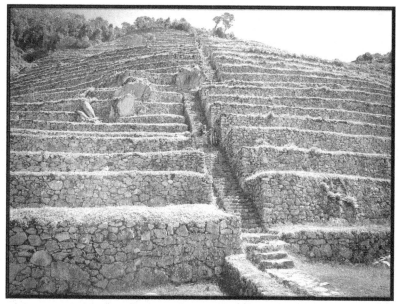

Nan and Pepe descend Intipata ruins
on the Inca Trail
(Photo by Doug Little)

Appreciating my relaxed pace, near the end of the four-day trek she asked to join me in my early departures. Just before the Sun Gate entrance into Machu Picchu we faced a particularly steep tier of steps, no more than 5 feet wide and inclined like a ladder. We felt we would be safer using both hands, unburdened by our poles, which we gave to a guide. She had consistently told me I was an inspiration, but it wasn't until we ascended the steps and she explained how she had spent her life fighting obesity and discrimination that I understood why facing challenges with courage and tenacity was so important to her. Near the top my companion froze, ashen and panting. I looked back at her, understanding right away that her panic was not only debilitating; it was potentially dangerous. I remembered what a panic attack looked like.

To ease her fears, I took a deep breath and told her I wanted to share a story about Rosie, my granddaughter. At a nearby playground two-year-old Rosie decided to climb a rope ladder that was probably beyond her ability, after which she intended to walk across another rope ladder while hanging on

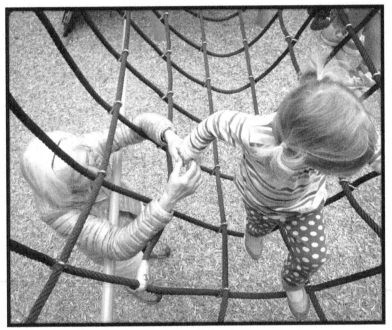

I can do this. Granddaughter Rosie
(Photo by Jodie Toft)

to ropes barely within her grasp. She insisted on trying. I stood below with arms outstretched, pretending I could catch her if she fell, and slowly coached her up the first ladder. She started across the horizontal ropes with her tiny fingers on one hand tightly grasping the stabilizing side rope and her other hand clutching my outstretched finger, moving so carefully from foothold to wobbly foothold muttering, *"I can do this. I can do this. I can do this."*

My anxious companion listened intently and nodded. Then, as we started up the steps, I could hear her soft voice behind me, "I can do this. I can do this. I can do this." At the top, she hugged me, tears streaming down our faces.

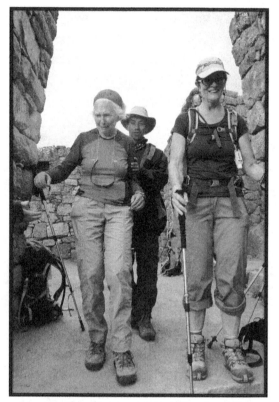

An emotional moment at the Sun Gate
entrance to Machu Picchu
(Photo by Doug Little)

For many people Machu Picchu is a holy place. As we trekked the Inca Trail, we explored in solitude archeological sites that seemed like practice versions of the grand Machu Picchu, all the while learning about the seamless social structure that mirrored the seamless placement of the rocks—rocks and spaces for light all aligned with the solstices, and all mimicking the shapes of the mountains in the distance.

It was easy to see why people think a special spirit inhabits the place. As an anthropologist, learning about patterns in the way of living, ruling, construction and harmony with space, time and the seasons enthralled me.

As a naturally nosy traveler, I was also interested in our porters, indigenous Quechua speaking Peruvians who ranged in age from their early twenties to early sixties. I seemed to be a source of endless amusement too, the white-haired grandma who carried her own pack in spite of her frozen shoulder. One day, frustrated by repeatedly catching my hair in my sunglasses, I determined to find a piece of string to hang my glasses around my neck. Since the only string I could find held up the toilet paper roll in our portable bathroom, I mimed what I wanted and why. After much confusion and a lot of chuckling, I had my string. Laughter, as well as love, has strong medicinal value.

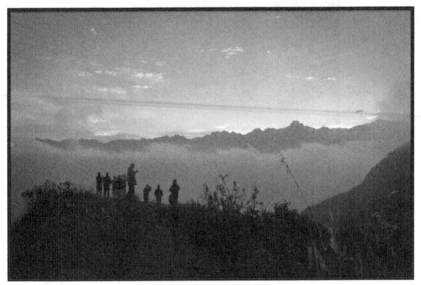

Sunrise breakfast over the Andes
along Inca Trail
(Photo by Doug Little)

Just before we crawled into our tents on our last night, our head guide asked if we wanted to see the sun rise over Machu Picchu. Of course! A knock on the tent at 5:00 a.m. alerted us to scramble into the darkness to climb the last rise overlooking Machu Picchu. Waiting to greet us, grinning with delight at our reactions, our porters offered steaming cups of coffee and tea.

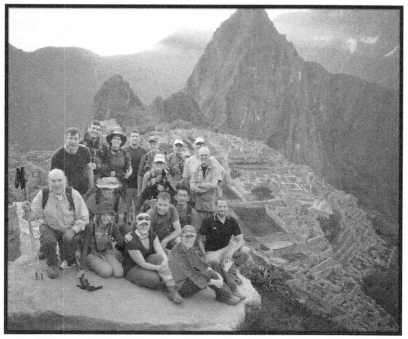

Group on way down from Sun Gate
into Machu Picchu

Before we left on the trek my daughter Jodie had sent an e-mail telling me I needed to complete two tasks while in Peru: drink some Peruvian beer (done) and learn a swear word in Quechua. The time had come to fulfill her second request. When I explained the challenge to our head guide and practical joker, Frances, his face exploded in incredulous astonished delight.

After pondering a few moments, eyes sparkling in the early morning light, he grinned and taught me to say *sakita muchai,* and then he walked me over to the youngest porter. I walked confidently to the young man, who giggled with excitement at being at the center of attention with the old woman. As all the other porters crowded around, sort of innocently, I smiled and said *sakita muchai* (Kiss my ass). All howled with laughter. Word quickly spread, more laughter .. the sun rose over Machu Picchu.

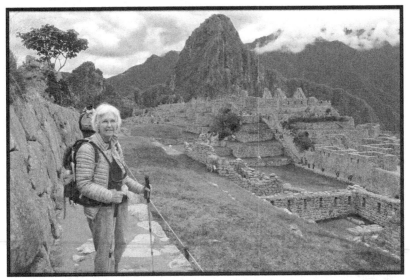

Nan at Machu Picchu
(Photo by Doug Little)

Chapter 28. Game Changers

Consistently at the top of my list of favorite annual events was the two-weeks we hosted at the Visitor's Center at The Nature Conservancy (TNC) Silver Creek Preserve at Picabo, Idaho. One of those responsible for creating this haven was Jack Hemingway. A lovely Hemingway memorial was a short walk on a path along the creek. Silver Creek, a blue ribbon fly-fishing site, is a fisherman's mecca. Humble pie graced the menu of even the best fisher-folk in the world when they came to the still, weedy gin-clear waters of Silver Creek, home to thousands of savvy trout that had perfected the art of flipping the middle fin.

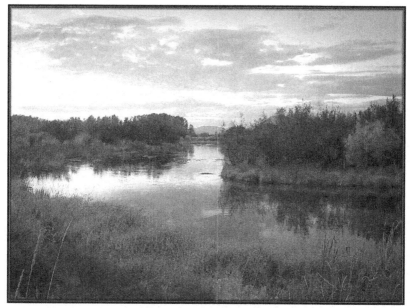

Silver Creek Preserve
(Photo by Doug Little)

The Nature Conservancy allowed people to volunteer as hosts at the Visitor's Center from early summer to the end of October, "working" several days each week and fishing or birding during their free time. Doug and I were fortunate enough to be in the right place at the right time one year to fill an open slot in the last two weeks of October, when the spawning brown trout moved into the waters, dug their redds and laid eggs. Since the role of host was renewable, not many opportunities appeared and we leapt at the chance.

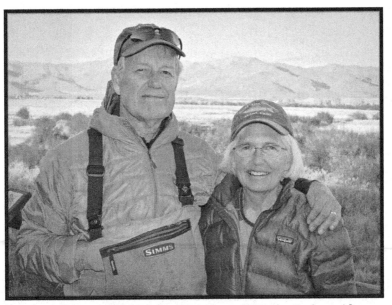

At Silver Creek (Photo courtesy of Kevin Erdman)]

Our job was to greet fishermen, make sure they signed in, sell hats and shirts, encourage donations, explain the history of the place and the rules, give advice on hatches and flies and complete at least one big project during our two weeks. One year we planted hundreds of young willows and aspen trees along the banks. Another year we sited and hung 70 birdhouses that had been built by another volunteer. We enjoyed helping young students frame and execute their projects, be it designing a boardwalk to allow handicapped access deep in the preserve or helping build a beaver lodge on a newly donated section of land. (Doug did most of the work. I helped a little.) TNC housed us in a cabin on the property, the starting point for my daily walk to the Visitor's Center with our dogs.

Since the Preserve is not conducive to road biking, I set up my bike and trainer on the front porch of the Center and rode for an hour nearly every day. Visitors invariably asked where I was going, when I would arrive, how fast I could ride on the porch, etc. etc. I think I heard it all. I generally asked if they were interested in knowing why I was cycling and some showed genuine interest in PFP, often asking for information for friends or family members who might find the program useful.

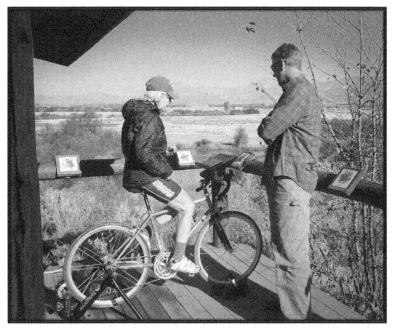

Testing Beneufit app at the Silver Creek
Visitors Center with Jeff Broderick
(Photo by Doug Little)

A few years ago a curious fisherman approached me as I was spinning away on the porch. He asked good questions about the efficacy of cycling for Parkinson's patients and wondered what I felt would be helpful beyond what I was doing already. I explained that I would like to keep an ongoing record of my progress. He wrote down my name and email before heading off to test his skill and luck with the trout.

Soon after I returned home I received a package from Jeff Broderick asking me to try out his product to see if it met my needs. I tried it, but it didn't help so I figured that was the end of that. Not so. Jeff designed another system for me to Beta test, which included monitoring heart rate and cadence as I tried to match the workout that had been specifically designed for me based on the PFP protocols and my personal data. I could see both current and historical results.

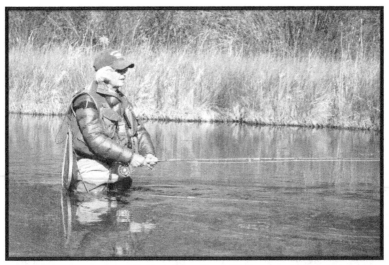

Forget PD. Just Fish.
(Photo courtesy of Kevin Erdman)

When Jeff contacted me in early October 2013 to see if he could bring a videographer to Seattle to record material for his website, I invited both of them to return to the starting place, Silver Creek, to make a video for his new company, Beneufit. I had never fished with a photographer shooting a movie over my shoulder. (I didn't catch anything until after they left.) Since I'm a compulsive person, trying to keep up with the Beneufit program and get a better fitness number each day was right up my alley. As with every intervention, I doubt it would work for everyone, but I found it another useful tool to keep me motivated. It also helped me begin to understand how my heart was responding to this intense cycling program.

♪ ♪ ♪ ♪ ♪

Miracles happened. At the World Parkinson's Congress in Montreal in the fall of 2013, I attended a lecture/class given by David Leventhal of Dance for PD, a program founded by him and John Heginbotham, principal dancers from the Marc Morris Dance Group, and the Brooklyn Parkinson Group in Brooklyn, New York. David astonished me with his ability to get 500 people sitting in rows, many with Parkinson's, dancing in place with abandon.

I knew I wanted to be part of this magic. The Northwest Parkinson's Foundation and Spectrum Dance Studio in Seattle sponsored Dance for PD classes in several locations, including one just a two-mile walk from our house. Never having danced in my life, I knew I would make a fool of myself in front of strangers and professional dancers. But, putting my pride in my pocket, in early January 2014 I took the awkward leap and began to dance, once each week for an hour and a half.

The Dance for PD program was anything but random. Each instructor was not only a professional dancer, but each had been trained extensively in realities of living with Parkinson's. Every class, every move in every class was based on needs of Parkinson's patients, beginning with the warm-ups and moving into dance sequences. Dancers started in our seats, learned increasingly complex hand and foot movements, then moved to the barre to extend flexibility by doing plies and finally, integrated all the moves into real dances, folk dances from around the world or portions of ballets.

As in the Pedaling For Parkinson's classes, and I imagine in all the other PD exercise programs, an important part of the experience was being with others who shared the same physical and cognitive challenges.   We spoke and moved the same language and we could laugh knowingly together. The

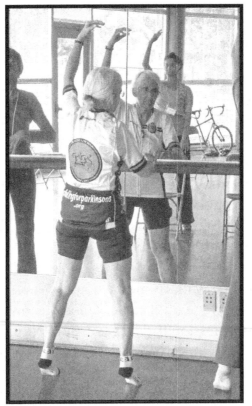

Dance for PD
program in Seattle
(Photo by Doug Little)

instructors never mentioned Parkinson's.   We were there to dance, not to wallow in disease, so we forgot about our disease, if only for ninety minutes each week, and became real dancers.

As I tried to follow the instructors, I pictured my own body looking just like theirs, gracefully executing complex hand and foot movements, even though a cursory glance in the mirror confirmed that my picture was pure fantasy. But it was a healthy fantasy. In my mind's eye, I was whole; a 34-year-old ballerina, not a 68-year-old PwP. I was free. I loved it.

By mid-March 2014 my frozen shoulder responded to the physical therapy, the biking, the medications and the dance. Again, as with my first experience with fast pace cycling back in 2009, the change happened rather suddenly. From my journal: "3/20 shoulder better for first time in 1.5 years; 4/8 shoulder better; 4/17 shoulder improving; 4/22 shoulder improving." As the range of motion in my shoulder improved, I began to regain the use of my right hand.

In mid-May I changed my drug regimen to Sinemet bolstered by 8mg of Requip XL. Soon I realized I could write my name, open jars, cut my food and type, albeit slowly, then more rapidly as the days passed. Tenacity, a belief that there were real answers out there for my Parkinson's and a willingness to try just about anything that made some sense paid off with another return toward health.

Chapter 29. RAGBRAI 2014: The Princess and the Frog

Doug and I considered riding RAGBRAI again. Due to the broken finger and frozen shoulder we had planned to ride a tandem but after a couple of painful practices, we were not sure. Once my shoulder healed Doug wondered if I thought I could ride my own solo bike again. I was willing to give it a try, knowing I could sag in the van if necessary.

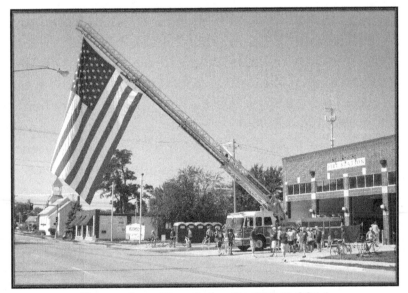

Fire station, Clear Lake, RAGBRAI 2014
(Photo by Doug Little)

Seven riders with PD rode in our group, John and Cidney from prior years along with Carol, Doug, Mike and Bill, all early onset but me. At 68 perhaps I was getting a little old for this adventure, but I figured I would do it as long as I could.

Sunday's ride started into headwinds that continued for most of the 80-mile ride. I felt fine. The next evening Jay spoke about his research and asked each of the PwPs to tell our story. Carol had been training for the ride on a tandem with her husband, not quite understanding the magnitude of what they were getting into, but was brave and game for the adventure. Bill was still really strong after 18 years with PD and Doug was looking at DBS after just a few years.

When we met him Saturday night, Mike frightened us all with his massive dystonia and dyskinesia. He was so overcome with wild random motions that none of us knew how he was going to make this trip. It was truly scary. After few days of steady cycling, when he was asked to tell his story, none of us could quite believe the man walking smoothly and confidently to the front of the room was the same man we had seen Saturday evening. Between cycling hard and closely monitoring his medication schedule, he was fine the rest of the week.

In 2014 the group had the benefit of an outstanding photographer determined to make an album of the trip. Leigh was particularly interested in action shots of PwPs. Fortunately he could turn around and take photos while riding at 15 miles an hour as long as his buddies were clearing the way.

On Wednesday night a reporter came to Jay's dog and pony show looking for a different take on RAGBRAI. She asked if she could speak with me after the presentation and I showed up on the evening and morning news, shaking hand and all.

The next day Leigh decided it was time for action photos of the group "celebrity" so on a picture perfect day I was treated like a princess. Leigh had two other cyclists form a wedge with me in the middle to clear other riders. Since I usually biked alone, this attention was pretty heady. I rode faster and with more authority than I ever did, smiling all the way. It felt silly but I knew I could get used to this!

When we finally arrived at our destination town, Waverly, we had no idea how to find the host house. With all phone circuits clogged, we would have to rely on locals to direct us, not generally a successful strategy. Looking across the street at the fire station we decided surely the firemen could tell us how to find the house. The three firemen discussed the issue for some time, trying to sort out a route that might be relatively flat and direct. Deciding we would be forced to make too many turns, they finally told us to just follow the fire truck, which we did, adding immeasurably to the Princess image. I knew in my heart this was too good to last.

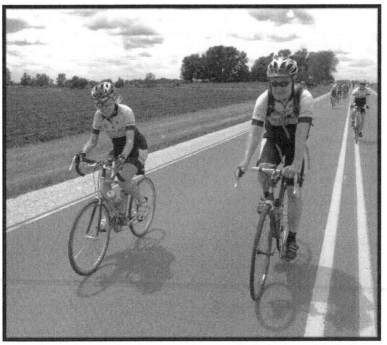

RAGBRAI 2014 (Photo courtesy of Leigh Atkins)

The next morning the sun had disappeared, replaced by an accurate forecast for falling temperatures, wind and heavy rain. Shortly, as our rain-soaked jackets stuck to our chilly bodies, all vision of a princess had melted away. Wind and rain brutally lashed us all. When Doug and I stopped at a school to get a second breakfast, he told me to wait for him inside the building. I joined about 2,000 cold, soaking wet riders crammed into the building built for no more than 500. A voice on the intercom told us the fire department said most of us had to leave. Shivering into a state of hypothermia, I was not about to move. I must have looked wretched. Strangers wrapped me in bubble wrap. A nice man asked apologetically if he could hold me in his arms to try to transfer some body heat. I stood in the hallway hugging a perfect stranger. Members of our team took me, shaking uncontrollably and turning blue, out of the drafty hallway into the cafeteria where a woman immediately gave up her seat.

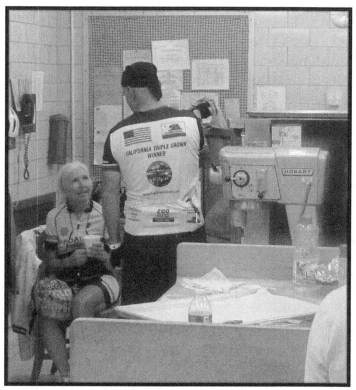

Nan in front of warming oven
(Photo by Doug Little)

Very soon a determined cook came out of the kitchen to fetch me. She put a chair in front of the warming oven and opened both doors, blasting me with dry heat. I finally had enough sense to remove my jacket, dry it, and then I swapped it for my shirt, which I dried in front of the oven. Princess to Freezing Frog. Ahhh, life's transitions in a heartbeat.

On the last night of RAGBRAI 2014, Independence, Iowa celebrated with bands and fireworks. Even our host nursing home joined the festivities with a band playing under canopies in the parking lot and residents lined up in their wheelchairs along the front of the building. As our group sat around in the mild evening breeze, reminiscing events of the week, it occurred to me that surely they would like to learn some steps from Dance for PD. PD members and a couple of others joined in. Carol discarded her cane and in moments the parking lot rang with laughter as we bobbled through plies and line dances, absurdly delighted.

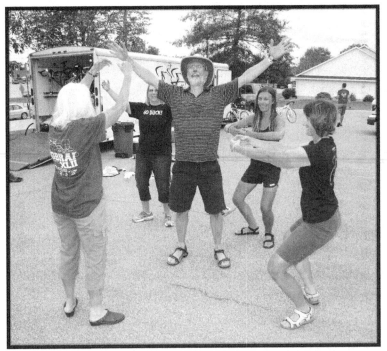

Dancing for PD at RAGBRAI 2014
(Photo by Doug Little)

Chapter 30. REM Again

My strategy for controlling the REM Sleep Behavior Disorder worked well until September 2014 when, the night before we left for a six week fishing and hiking trip in the Canadian Rockies, through Montana and back to Silver Creek, I dreamed that the same woman who had visited at the time of my mother's memorial showed up again, ready to hurt me again. I yelled at her to leave me alone, then swung my left leg back and kicked as hard as I could, right into the small chest of drawers next to the bed.

Although I knew I had injured myself, we were all packed to head east in the morning to join our son Jason and his family at a football game before heading to Canada. I realized that if we went to the hospital, we would miss the game and the doctors would just take x-rays, tape the (likely) broken toe and admonish me to wear hard tip shoes and take it easy. Feeling confident in my self-diagnosis, I took another half sleeping pill and finished the night in bed. To protect my broken toe, I wore either my stiff hiking boots or my fishing boots for most of the next six weeks. An x-ray taken the day after we returned showed a white line where I had broken the middle toe in half from the tip to the foot; it had healed nicely. The doctor told me that smashing my big toe would likely accelerate the arthritis already present but that was just part of life. (Our team won the football game.)

I finally resolved the conflict with my night visitor when I owned the problem as mine. People with bubble wrap and warming ovens would not be there for me in every crisis; I had to make the most of my own inner resources if I were to successfully live with Parkinson's.

♪ ♪ ♪ ♪ ♪

The Burgess Shale in SE British Columbia is the most extensive pre-Cambrian fossil record in the world. Although the name, Burgess Shale, registered a small ding in my memory, it never made the trip on to my bucket list. However, since we were within striking distance, a mere 17-mile hike, it would seem silly to miss the opportunity, with or without a broken toe and Parkinson's. Due to the fragile nature of fossils and danger posed by poachers, access to this world heritage site was limited to ranger guided hikes.

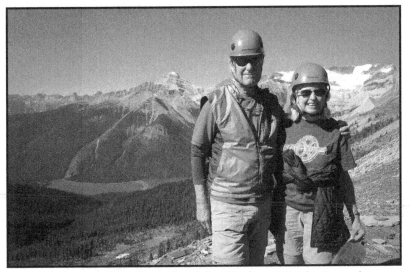

At the Burgess Shale in Yoho National Park, Canada

We decided if we told the ranger that I had Parkinson's and probably a broken toe, we would be denied the opportunity to hike to the fossil beds. We kept our mouths shut and looked over the rest of the climbing party to see if, in fact, I would be bringing up the rear. The others looked plenty fit. Clearly the ranger wanted to hustle us along. I did my best but inevitably slowed the pace of the group. At one rest point she pointed out that the next section was a little flatter and wondered if perhaps I could speed up a bit. I assured her I would do my best. That day my Fitbit recorded 41,492 steps, 292 flights of stairs, 17.04 miles. It was a special hike, partly because I didn't think I could do it or was sure I even wanted to try. But I did and we were both happy and exhausted. (I found a 3 inch trilobite, perfectly preserved for 505 MILLION years with even its eye intact!)

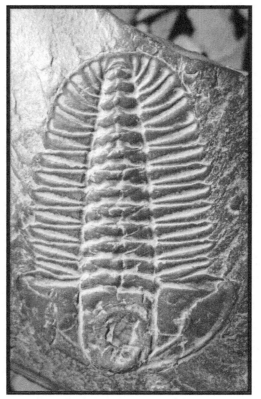

Burgess Shale Trilobite
(Photo by Doug Little)

Chapter 31. Advocacy

We can be part of the parade or we can cheer as the marchers go by. Either way we add something to the mix. When Jay had first suggested that we ride across Iowa, I hadn't taken into account that as I rode people would ask about my jersey and about Pedaling For Parkinson's and that I would be expected to know something about the disease and what people were doing about it. Fortunately, I had an excellent teacher in Jay and in my first RAGBRAI in 2009 I learned a great deal about the disease and what I should expect for myself and for others.

The science intrigued me—more accurately, the paucity of knowledge about what Parkinson's actually is, how one gets it, and why some strategies mediate symptoms. Although I'm sure it's not the last frontier (I'm quite sure there will always be frontiers) it helped me emotionally to step back and use my intellect to learn what was going on in my deteriorating Parkinson's brain.

When I realized how little was actually known, it was not a big step to move into advocacy. Due to the rides across Iowa, and certainly the climb of Mount Kilimanjaro, I developed enough of a reputation that I was asked to speak in various venues. From those speaking engagements I learned what people wanted to know, both PwPs and professionals in the field. I had plenty of homework to do before I was even minimally competent to answer questions. Of course, I did not give medical advice. I just told my stories.

When I saw a blurb about an open position on the People with Parkinson's Advisory Council (PPAC) of the national Parkinson's Disease Foundation (PDF), it seemed like a good idea to apply (though I had no idea of the range of work being done by PDF or what would be expected of me as a member of PPAC).

Although I knew I should always clarify expectations before jumping in, if a role sounded interesting I applied for it, and often figured it out as I went along.

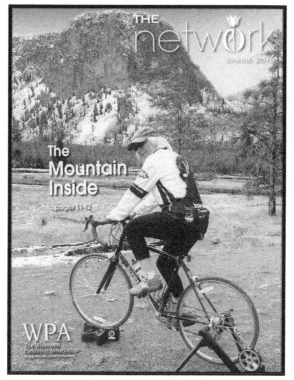

Advocacy event for the
Wisconsin Parkinson Association,
The Network, Spring 2013

Our job as PPAC members was to advise the PDF Board of Directors and staff on proposed directions and programs, ensuring that the patient's perspective was represented in the programs and actions of the organization. As a member of PPAC I would attend two meetings in New York City each year as well as participate in monthly calls. Each year the spring meeting coincided with the Parkinson's Unity Walk in Central Park, a fundraiser for seven Parkinson's organizations including

PDF, which provided an opportunity to meet national movers and shakers in the Parkinson's arena. As I was still newly diagnosed, I had much to learn, including that PDF is one of the premier Parkinson's organizations in the world. It was an honor to be selected as a member of PPAC.

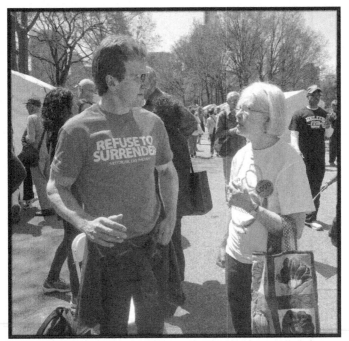

Unity Walk in Central Park with Davis Phinney
(Photo by Doug Little)

I tend to think of PDF as synonymous with "leadership"; it's the prow of an icebreaker, opening new routes to research, and new routes to serve and educate. By identifying promising leads and giving startup grants to people with creative ideas, PDF often initiates collaborations that lead to important insights and discoveries.

PPAC is a collaborative unit. From members I have learned about global projects and research opportunities at the National Institutes of Health and Johns Hopkins University. PDF arranged a PPAC meeting at the World Parkinson's Congress in

2013 in Montreal, further expanding my knowledge and horizons, thereby enhancing my ability to advocate.

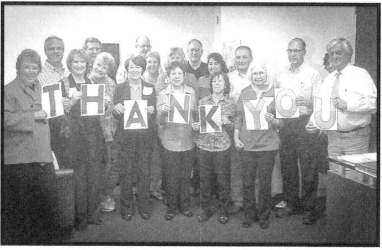

People with Parkinson's Advisory Council to PDF
April 2014

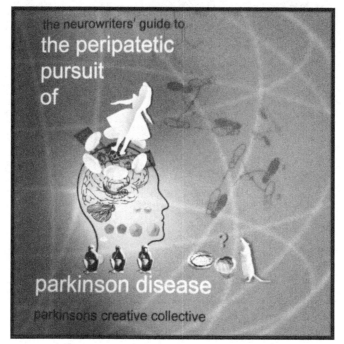

Support group between two covers
by the Parkinson's Creative Collective

Another important voice in the Parkinson's community is the Parkinson's Creative Collective (PCC), people who met one another online at the NeuroTalk PD forum and, deciding that PwPs needed a support group for themselves, their caregivers, and people in the broader neurology community, created the book *The Peripatetic Pursuit of Parkinson Disease*. Over the four-year course of producing the book, two of the eleven authors died, leaving a legacy matched by few. I was asked to join the Board of Directors of PCC, again introducing me to some of the finest advocates who happen to be PwPs.

Professional cyclist Glenn Erickson, who was diagnosed with PD when I was, organized a fundraising ride to help with Parkinson's in the northwest by supporting an expansion plan for Pedaling For Parkinson's. This turned into an annual event.

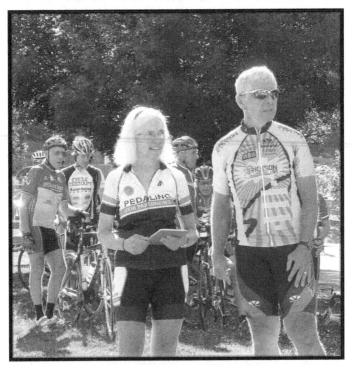

With Glenn Erickson at his
August 2014 fundraising ride
(Photo by Doug Little)

Although primarily focused on research, massive levels of research, the Michael J. Fox Foundation launched a new educational program, Partners in Parkinson's (PiP) directed particularly at PwPs who did not yet receive services. MJFF asked me to be an ambassador while they got PiP up and running.

The Northwest Parkinson's Foundation asked me to join them in Washington DC for the Parkinson's Action Network (PAN) conference as a delegate from Washington State trying to educate politicians and their staff on issues related to PD.

I never knew when the next advocacy door would open, but based on my past history, chances were good I would walk on in. Like the people from PCC, I am also interested in leaving a legacy, whether it is as grand as their book or as straightforward as helping people get on bicycles.

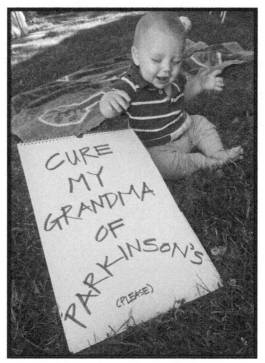

Grandson Levi as advocate
(Photograph courtesy of Jodie Toft)

As long as I maintain courage and tenacity and I'm surrounded by love, I'll be okay. I can't do a whole lot of things, but I'm learning to dance. . .

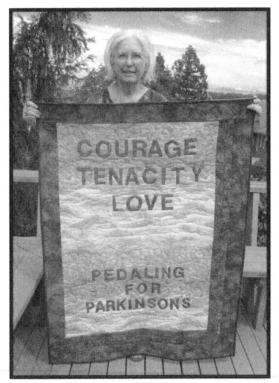

Courage Tenacity Love
(Photo by Doug Little)

Chapter 32. Epilogue

After not hearing from Joe DiIenno, our psychiatrist friend, since shortly after being diagnosed, in early September 2014 I received a letter from him. We had run into a colleague of his at the World Parkinson's Congress in Montreal and had asked him to convey our best wishes. Joe contacted me a year later with insights that I believe apply to all PwPs. He gave permission to quote from his letter here.

September 2014

Dear Nan,

I hope this note comes at a suitable time for you and Doug.

Friendship, however distant, is always gratifying to me.

As you know, all journeys outward are journeys inward.

From our being together those years ago, I know you realize that Parkinson's Disease is a thing. Whatever meaning it has in your life is what counts—not the disease itself. Disease is a way of thinking about the challenges <u>in your life</u> and it is not about the limits it presents. What exists is the person—Nan, incidentally with whatever limitations and capacities are present. How you choose to respond to life matters—the inward journey is about choice. What does exist is Nan—wonderful, simply wonderful.

Parkinson's is a vicarious disease, uncontrolled and very inconvenient at times: the constancy of youth in yourself, the reliable resilience of your self-determination, the continuous love of your life—these do not waiver. The beauty of your character is so grand as to make any such inconvenience trite.

So it is not that the treatment works, but that you make the treatment and it works for you. It is always the person and the person's choice of a full life that makes one's life one's own. Circumstances, even the circumstances of one's own body, do not have to interfere with the courage of self-determination nor with loving others. Handling challenges, choosing effectively to live a full life—Nan's way—is what comes to mind when I think of you and Doug.

Friendship is one of the fulfillments of my life. Engaging each person I encounter adds mystery, wonder and love, deepens understanding and frequently eventuates in friendship—as with us. I have in a way travelled many lives. I live the blessings of many friendships. You and Doug in particular are rewarding to know.

Thank God for all he has given us and God bless you.

Joe

Acknowledgments

A high school friend wrote a poem that captures how I feel about sharing the stories in this book:

I give you all my treasures in a brown paper sack.
About your feet I lay them.
Step softly.
It is my heart.

--Elizabeth Wissman

Writing is essentially a lonely endeavor but neither the story nor the telling would be possible without the real and virtual banners of encouragement that wrap around my life.

From the very beginning and through each day my husband, Doug, has looked this disease straight in the eye and refused to flinch. Our children, Jason and Jodie, and their spouses, Christy Kirchner and Jason Toft, support my every endeavor with clear observations and helpful actions. Each family has added two grandchildren: Aiden and Ryan, Rosie and Levi who, in addition to making me laugh, give me ample reason to do my best to be mobile and whineless.

My older brothers, Tom and Bob, constantly express amazement at anything and everything I do. No strangers to either advocacy or people in pain, they give their full measure of love and appreciation, as do Doug's sister Ann and half-sister Lynne.

Community builders who do not have PD protect me from the isolation that can easily swallow PwPs. Each member of my hiking group, the DAWGS, accepts me as I am, notwithstanding limitations, as do the sheepish members of

Doug's group, the Torrs. The Dance for PD troupe has an unspoken supportive bond, facilitated by our expert leaders.

YMCAs in the US and abroad throw their hearts into the Pedaling For Parkinson's program, encouraging me to continue my efforts by providing opportunities for other patients to do the same. Each call I get confirms my sense of self-worth, which at times wanes when I sit in solitude. Glenn Erickson, his wife Nancy, and the selfless cyclists who put on the Glenn Erickson PFP annual fundraising ride continually make me shake my head in wonderment. Our neighborhood book club spends more time supporting each other than on literary endeavors, with Diann Shope generously sharing her writing experience. Webs of community networks sustain us all.

Members of PPAC candidly speak up for people with Parkinson's, not hesitating to challenge each other's assumptions or interpretations, ensuring honesty instead of self-pity.

The members of the Parkinson's Creative Collective (PCC) make the best of every day and every opportunity, always pushing the envelope and each other, in no small part to honor those who came before. Many thoughtful, intelligent, inquiring (and skeptical) people post on the NeuroTalk site, offer ideas, sympathy, and support as well as themselves as lab rats to test new ideas.

Without Jay Alberts, Ph.D., the kinesthesiologist and neuroscientist who recognized the correlation between high cadence cycling and mitigation of Parkinson's symptoms, I expect I would be sitting in a wheelchair or certainly using a cane by this time. The entire trajectory of my life and my disease changed because of Jay.

Drs. John Roberts and Laird Patterson answer my every question, generally within 24 hours. They each spoke of the value of exercise at our first meetings and have been relentless in touting its efficacy for all who can do it, even a little bit.

Where Jay's insights affected my physical wellbeing, Joe DiIenno reached into my soul.

Nudging me along, gently but persistently, have been retired editor, Phyllis Hatfield, and an old friend turned editor from our children's school days, Kathy Bradley, whose knowledge of the Chicago Manual of Style continues to astonish me. At each tough turn, Kathy offered suggestions that helped clarify both my thinking and my writing.

Susie Weber shared her artistic gifts unstintingly. I never imagined that this fellow Kilimanjaro climber who quietly lives with MS would keep entering my life in such wonderful ways. As with Brandis Gunderson, whose friendship that began on Kilimanjaro grew so strong that she feels like a surrogate daughter.

Photographers Jeff Rennicke, Nathan Henwood, Kevin Erdman, Richard Baccus, Leigh Atkins and Grant Gunderson gave selflessly of their time and talents to support the project.

Each time we travel to Yellowstone and Silver Creek we anticipate renewing friendships with those who teach us, cheer us on and focus on something other than disease. You all recognize yourselves, quilting, catching fish and looking for lollipop trees in the forests. Jeff Broderick's relentless pursuit of something that works for PD patients offers insight into his character of commitment.

Friends from hikes and rides hold a special place on my virtual banner, from Ines and others who stayed with me much of the night on Kilimanjaro, to Dr. Jan who faithfully assumed the role of food cutter when I couldn't hold a knife during the Machu Picchu climb, to those who wrapped me in bubble wrap when I was near hypothermia on RAGBRAI and all those in between.

It has been my privilege to work with Native American students, TAs and elders from many tribes who taught me values of listening carefully and assuming little and who continue to be part of my life. I am honored by your friendship.

Although I have missed thanking many individuals, know that your encouragement and unfettered support mean everything.

To all who inspire me with your courage, tenacity and love, I thank you.

Appendix A: Pedaling For Parkinson's Protocols

✓ 3 times per week

✓ 1 hour each time
- 10 minutes warm up
- 40 minutes at 80-90 rpm
- 10 minutes cool down

✓ 60-85% of Maximum Heart Rate (MHR = roughly 220 minus your age)

While high cadence pedaling does not cure or stop the progression of PD, there is compelling evidence to show that it does make a real difference in symptoms for most who try it. It's changing the lives of increasing numbers of participants who, before PFP, depended on medication and eventually surgery to cope with the effects of PD. Note that PFP is not intended as a substitute for prescribed medications.

Appendix B: Research Studies

- 11/2009—Signed up for Washington Parkinson Disease Registry
- 4/2010—Signed up for Pacific Northwest Udall Center (PANUC) for studies of causes of cognitive impairment
- 6/2010—Joined the VA Alzheimer's Disease Research Center
- 6/2010—Participated in a small study to investigate control of hand movements
- 7/2012—Genetic Characterization of Movement Disorders, NIH/NIA
- 9/2012—Entered the PANUC Clinical Core and Data Management Continuing Study
- 11/2012—Parkinson's Genetic Research (PaGeR) Study for genetic research to identify genes that increase a person's risk of getting PD and/or developing cognitive problems
- 2/2013—Galantamine drug study to determine whether fMRI can identify which patients with PD will respond well to the acetylcholine replacement medication
- 5/2013—Enrolled in NIH Clinical Center, which conducts biomedical research concerning health and disease
- 5/2013—Imaging Biomarkers in Parkinson's Disease, NIH
- 6/2013—PANUC provides education, investigates causes of cognitive impairment, and shares results with the community (continuing program)
- 10/13—PaGeR study to find genes that increase the likelihood of developing certain PD related problems, such as difficulties with thinking and memory, VA and NIH

- 10/2013—MARK-PD study to identify Biomarkers for Parkinson disease and PD related cognitive impairment, Johns Hopkins/NINDS
- 11/2013—PANUC Galantamine study to be able to link data from MRI brain imaging and CSF markers
- 3/2014—P-DIGeST Parkinson's Disease Gut Study
- 11/2014—Haptoglobin Phenotype and Smoking: study Effects on Iron Levels in Parkinson's disease through MRI Study, Bastyr University
- 2/2015—Telemedicine Study to test the efficacy of using telemedicine to provide accurate diagnosis and treatment for rural patients, University of Rochester, New York
- 3/2015—mPower (Mobile Parkinson Observatory for Worldwide, Evidence-based Research); Parkinson Disease iOS usability study to determine how to use remote devices to collect continuous data, Sage Bionetworks
- 5/2015—Physiological Studies of Movement Disorders to better understand how the brain controls movement, learn more about movement disorders and train movement disorder specialists, NIH

Bibliography

Resources Cited in the Text

Parkinsons Creative Collective. *The Peripatetic Pursuit of Parkinson Disease.* Little Rock: Parkinsons Creative Collective, 2013.

Schneider, Lori. *More Than a Mountain: Our Leap of Faith.* USA: Empowerment Through Adventure, 2012.

White, Richard. *Remembering Ahanagran: Storytelling in a Family's Past.* New York: Hill & Wang, 1998.

Books for PwPs, Their Loved Ones and Caregivers

Fox, Michael J. *Always Looking Up: The Adventures of an Incurable Optimist.* New York: Hyperion, 2009.

Fox, Michael J. *Lucky Man: A Memoir.* New York: Hyperion, 2002.

Lieberman, Abraham. *The Muhammad Ali Parkinson Center 100 Questions & Answers About Parkinson Disease.* Sudbury, MA: Jones and Bartlett Learning, 2011.

Mischley, Laurie K. *Natural Therapies for Parkinson's Disease.* Seattle: Coffeetown Press, 2010.

Newsom, Hal. *H.O.P.E.: Four Keys to a Better Quality of Life for Parkinson's People.* Seattle: Northwest Parkinson's Foundation, 2006.

Parkinsons Creative Collective. *The Peripatetic Pursuit of Parkinson Disease.* Little Rock: Parkinsons Creative Collective, 2013

Phinney, Davis. *The Happiness of Pursuit: A Father's Courage, a Son's Love and Life's Steepest Climb.* Boston: Houghton Mifflin Harcourt, 2011

Robb, Karl. *A Soft Voice in a Noisy World: A Guide to Dealing and Healing with Parkinson's Disease.* USA: RobbWorks, 2012.

Schneider, Lori. *More Than A Mountain: Our Leap of Faith.* USA: Empowerment Through Adventure 2012.

Key Organizations and Websites Serving the PD Community

American Parkinson Disease Association Foundation. Its mission is to ease the burden and find the cure. http://www.apdaparkinson.org

HealthUnlocked. A social network for health. London: HealthUnlocked. https://healthunlocked.com/

Michael J. Fox Foundation for Parkinson's Research. The foundation (MJFF) is dedicated to finding a cure for Parkinson's disease through an aggressively funded research agenda and to ensuring the development of improved therapies for those living with Parkinson's today. New York: Michael J. Fox Foundation. https://www.michaeljfox.org/

National Institute of Neurological Disorders and Stroke. The institute (NINDS) conducts and supports research on brain and nervous system disorders. Bethesda, MD: National Institute of Neurological Disorders and Stroke. http://www.ninds.nih.gov/

NeuroTalk Support Groups. Support groups for neurological brain disorders, including Parkinson's Disease. Newburyport, MA: Psych Central. http://neurotalk.psychcentral.com/

The Northwest Parkinson's Foundation (NWPF). The only independent regional Parkinson's organization serving Washington State. NWPF aims to establish optimal quality of life for the Northwest Parkinson's community through awareness, education, advocacy and care. http://nwpf.org

Parkinson's Action Network. The one organization in Washington, DC, advocating for better treatments and a cure on behalf of the entire Parkinson's community. Washington, DC: Parkinson's Action Network (PAN). http://www.parkinsonsaction.org/

Parkinson's Disease Foundation and the PDF Resource List. The list provides information about organizations, books and websites that can help you live with PD. New York: Parkinson's Disease Foundation. http://www.pdf.org/resourcelink

Pedaling For Parkinson's. An organization (PFP) committed to advancing our understanding of how physical activity impacts the motor symptoms associated with Parkinson's Disease. Chagrin Falls, OH: Pedaling For Parkinson's. http://www.pedalingforparkinsons.org/

Other Organizations and Websites

Multiple organizations and websites serve the PD community. Many are listed in the back of the book *Peripatetic Pursuit of Parkinson Disease.* They cover these categories:

Alternative Treatments

Caregivers

Clinical Trials

Deep Brain Stimulation

Drug Development

Environmental Issues

Especially for the Newly Diagnosed

Exercise

Hospitals

Legal Issues

Living with PD: Books by PwPs

Medical Guides

National and International Organizations

Non-Motor Symptoms

Nutrition

Patient-Centered Medicine and Orgs

Patient-Led and Patient-Centric Groups

Resource List

Sham Surgery

Therapies

Traditional Eastern Medicine

Work and Disability Issues

About The Author

Diagnosed with Parkinson's disease in early 2008 at age 62, Nan Little is a wife, grandma, sibling, teacher, volunteer, writer, speaker and Parkinson's advocate. Generally controlling her symptoms through high cadence cycling, she rode across Iowa in RAGBRAI in 2009, 2010, 2012 and 2014, climbed Mt. Kilimanjaro in 2011, trekked to the Annapurna Base Camp in Nepal in 2012, and hiked the Inca Trail to Machu Picchu in Peru in 2013.

Nan holds a bachelor's degree in English and Spanish from Albion College and a Ph.D. in Anthropology from the University of Washington where she worked with Native American tribes preparing students for success in science and math at the university level.

She represents Pedaling For Parkinson's, serves on the Parkinson's Disease Foundation's (PDF) People with Parkinson's Advisory Council (PPAC), is a member of the board of the Parkinson Creative Collective and is an advisor for Beneufit, a company that makes an assistive cycling app for people with Parkinson's.

Nan can be contacted at nan.little@comcast.net
Her website is: www.nanlittle.com